SUSAN K. DELAINE

Foreword by Dr. Peter Bauth

INTRODUCTION BY REBECCA PEABODY ESTEPP

THE AUTISM COOKBOOK

101 GLUTEN-FREE AND DAIRY-FREE RECIPES

Skyhorse Publishing

www.skyhorsepublishing.com

10 9 8 7 6 5 4 3 2 1

Library of Congress Cataloging-in-Publication Data is available on file.
ISBN: 978-1-61608-019-8

Printed in China

This book is intended to be a resource for autism information and recipes. It is not intended to prevent, diagnose, treat or cure any condition or to provide medical advice. Consult a health or medical professional prior to making dietary changes.

Contents

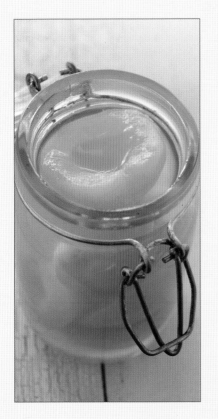

Author's note

The title of this book expresses the purpose for which it is written. My intention is for you to experience joy and ease in your gluten free/casein free (GFCF) journey with your loved one. I have come to find that the key to great GFCF cooking lies in relaxing and enjoying the experience. Don't worry—everything else will flow.

Chances are you have found this book because someone you love has autism, ADHD, ADD, or a similar developmental condition. You are interested in a biomedical approach to helping the person gain wellness in his or her body, yielding improvements in behavior, focus, attention, and physical comfort. You realize removing offensive foods is one major part of the health approach—and this is a general truth in wellness.

Our son, Justin, was diagnosed with autism at the age of three. Within three weeks of changing his diet, we began to see drastic improvements in his sleep, mood, and language. We were convinced that a GFCF diet for children like Justin was more of a health necessity than a choice.

How is this so? Most children with autism cannot digest gluten and casein, a condition called food sensitivity or intolerance. The simple truth is that undigested food builds up in the digestive tract and wreaks havoc on all body systems, including the brain. Thus, food affects behavior.

Please visit the recommended Web sites listed on page 236 to further your understanding of cooking GFCF. If you are convinced and want to learn more it will be very easy to find grocers, health professionals, educators, family members, and friends who will support you in your journey. Most importantly, remember your true purpose for seeking a GFCF diet and worry less about making perfectly round pancakes. If your first batch is misshapen, cut it up, dip it in maple syrup, and share it with someone you love!

Foreword

Health and wellness is all about addressing and correcting the cause; headaches do not result from a lack of Aspirin. Indigestion is not a result from a lack of Pepcid. Depression is not a result of a lack of Wellbutrin, and autism is certainly not a condition resulting from a lack of medication. Autism has, as its origins, an imbalance of normal physiology. Addressing this aberrant physiology should be every parent's first impulse.

There are many ways to do this. However, with closer consideration, only a few approaches address the primary and the determining causes; the determining being chemical toxicity, physical traumatism, and emotional tendencies or stressors that lead to these aberrant functions; and the primary being the actual manifestation of these stressors, brain hemispheric deficiency, nutritional deficiency sublaxation complex, and heavy metal toxicity.

For years now, clinicians and researchers have noticed positive changes in the physical and emotional health of children under chiropractic care, for example. Among the observed benefits are improvements in children with hyperactivity, autism, anxiety, low mental stamina, lack of concentration, asthma, and discipline problems. Improvement in grades and IQ has also been recorded.

Combine this now with the overwhelming body of evidence that shows direct connections between specific nutritional deficiencies and cognitive health and development issues and one begins to see a positive paradigm shift emerging in healthcare and the standard treatment of these childhood conditions, such as autism—treatments that have, until recently, been largely ineffective.

In my practice and in the practice of many colleagues, care is given based on this different paradigm of health and the results are nothing short of extraordinary. Give the information in this book a diligent try—you have nothing to lose and so very, very much to gain.

—Dr. Peter Bauth, D.C. LCP,
Trilogy Wellness

Introduction

January 1, 2001 was "D-Day" for my family. No, we did not storm the beaches of Normandy, although at times I felt so challenged that it did seem akin to a war. In reality, our D-Day was different. The "D" stood for diet. It was on that day that my husband and I started our almost three-year-old son, Eric, on the Gluten Free Casein Free (GFCF) diet.

Eric was diagnosed with autism in November of 2000. We were given a grim prognosis by our pediatrician. I also remember having an overwhelming feeling that this trusted pediatrician knew nothing about autism and knew nothing of my son or my family.

Luckily, I found a great network of parents on the internet that were treating their children's symptoms through diet and supplements following the Defeat Autism Now (DAN) protocol. The GFCF diet was central to this treatment. Due to my son's bowel problems (alternating constipation and diarrhea) a diet made perfect sense to me.

My trusted group of veteran internet parents, who would later be the individuals to start Talk About Curing Autism (TACA), gave me guidance through the early days of GFCF. There was not much available to purchase at my local grocery store so I took many trips to health food stores. I bought some items online and learned to cook like my Scottish grandmother—meat and potatoes for almost every dinner.

A short time later, Eric started to respond to the diet. The first improvement was the cessation of his night screaming. After that, Eric's mystery fevers disappeared. And then a miracle happened— Eric started to behave much better than before the diet. I have to believe that it was simply because he felt better. Let's face it; all of us do better when we feel well.

My son is now thriving. He will be twelve in a few short weeks. I still classify him as a child with autism, although we have a few opinions from teachers and therapists that he doesn't meet the qualification for autism any longer, which shows fantastic progress. I know that the GFCF diet was the foundation for his improved state and could not have been attained unless we went through our diet "D-Day" so long ago.

—Rebecca Peabody Estepp, National Manager, TACA (Talk About Curing Autism)

Autism and Diet

Autism currently affects one in ninety-one persons. Some signs of autism may appear during infancy. Other children develop normally and regress sharply between the ages of eighteen months to two years. The set of symptoms in autism will differ from person to person. Because symptoms range from very minor to very severe, autism is considered to be a "spectrum" disorder.

Research has shown that many autistic children have damaged intestinal tracts resulting from an overgrowth of bacteria. Some children are born with this condition. Other children are born with healthy digestive tracts and experience damage when exposed to environmental poisons, medications, processed and contaminated foods, and other toxins in our world. This damage can result in "food sensitivity" or "food intolerance," a condition in which the intestines cannot fully digest certain foods. Three common food sensitivity culprits are gluten (from wheat, barley, rye, and oat), casein (from cow's milk and goat's milk), and soy. Particles of foods left undigested in the intestine leak into the blood stream and have an adverse effect on the brain. This effect, similar to that of opiate drugs, can cause impairments in speech, motor skills, mood, focus, and learning and can worsen existing challenges. A diet free from gluten, casein, and soy (GFCFSF) can alleviate the discomfort a child is experiencing.

Like my son, Justin, many autistic children also have food allergies. A food allergy is a condition of the immune system in which the body "fights" against foods it believes to be harmful. This book is exclusive of common food sensitivity culprits (gluten, casein, and soy) as well as some of the most common food allergens (wheat, rice, egg, milk, peanut, tree nuts, fish, and shellfish).

The GFCFSF diet is the most common type of autism diet and is the focus of this book. However, there are other specific diets that can be used to meet the child's needs. It is helpful to work with a supportive healthcare professional who will provide testing, over time, to determine if your child's diet approach is working. Other diets include:

GFCFSF: Gluten Free, Casein Free, Soy Free

GFCF: Gluten Free, Casein Free

Specific Carbohydrate: A diet free from gluten, all starches (potato, corn, rice, all grains), and sugars. The diet allows specially cultured dairy products to be consumed. The goal of this diet is to stop the growth of microbes by eliminating foods that feed them.

Feingold Diet: Pinpoint and completely eliminate sensitivity culprits, allergens, chemicals, additives, and salicylates. These offending items are eliminated from both the diet and the environment (e.g., lotions, soaps, toothpaste, medicines, household products).

Elimination Diet: This diet is based on eliminating all major food allergen and sensitivity culprits, eating free-range meats, specific fruits and vegetables, and rice-based milk and pastas. Its purpose is to identify and eliminate food culprits and reintroduce them gradually over a specified schedule. Elimination diets require close record-keeping of foods in correlation to behaviors.

Diet alone does not cure autism but removing offensive foods is one major portion of the healing process. To maximize the benefits of a GFCF diet, one should also take steps to heal the intestinal tract, support the immune system, and nurture the whole child through healing arts.

Why Raw?

This book features twenty-three raw recipes. Foods are considered to be "raw" if they have not been cooked above 118°F. A diet high in unprocessed, raw foods is a vital part of proper digestion and good health, and this is true for everyone. Raw foods contain their own enzymes to help us digest with ease, without over-taxing the body. Because raw foods are so easy to digest, they are detoxifying, highly nutritious, and give a boost to the immune system. These are added benefits for everyone, especially for those with autism or allergies.

I do not recommend consuming raw eggs, meat, or fish. Rather, in this book you will find several raw recipes using fruits, vegetables, seeds, herbs, and cold-pressed oils. Raw foods can be eaten in their natural state or they can be prepared into recipes to satisfy your texture and flavor preferences. In my family's experience, adding one raw item to each meal every day (either a prepared raw dish or a side of raw fruits, vegetables, or seeds) has a great cumulative effect!

For those who have temperature preferences, raw foods can be heated up to 118°F or chilled while keeping their enzymes and nutrients intact. Our son, Justin, finds it easier to chew certain textures of foods that are at room temperature or warmed slightly. Use a food thermometer to heat raw foods safely.

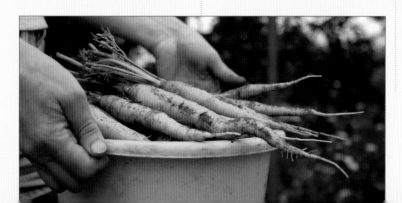

Going Organic

Organic fruits, vegetables, and other crops have been grown without the use of artificial pesticides, fertilizers, or Genetically Modified Organisms (GMOs). Organic animals have been raised without the use of antibiotics or growth hormones and have been fed an organic crop diet. In most cases, organic animals being raised for food are uncaged and allowed to roam freely. Therefore, they are leaner, stronger, and naturally disease-free. Because organic foods contain minimal additives, they maintain a natural state and are much easier to digest than non-organic foods.

The U.S. Department of Agriculture (USDA) has established standards for allowing foods to be labeled as "USDA Organic." Individual organic farmers who wish to use the USDA Organic label must meet these standards and undergo yearly inspections to assure compliance. There are three types of USDA Organic products:

100% Organic (the food label is allowed to display the "USDA Organic" symbol)

Organic (at least 95 percent of the ingredients are organic)

Made with Organic Ingredients (70 percent of the ingredients are organic; 30 percent contain no GMOs).

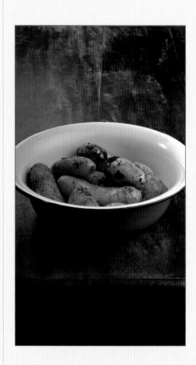

Replacements

USE…	INSTEAD OF…	FOR…
Quinoa or Buckwheat	Wheat Barley Rice Oat	Side dish Baking
Corn	Wheat Rice	Whole grain baking Cereal baking/frying Pasta
Baking soda Baking powder (aluminum-free)	Egg	Leavening in baking
Potato flour	Wheat Rice	Breading/frying and thickening
Potato	Rice	Side dish
Applesauce Water	Milks (cow's, rice, and soy)	Moisture in baking
Canola oil Corn oil Olive oil (cold-pressed oils are best)	Butter "Vegetable" oil (usually another name for soybean oil)	Frying and sautéing Moisture Dressings
Flax seed Sesame	Peanut Tree nuts Soy nut	"Nutty" flavoring Alternative to nut butters
Ginger, sesame, and garlic combined	Soy sauce	Flavor in Asian dishes
Honey Agave nectar Evaporated cane juice Xylitol	White granulated sugar	Sweetening

Guide to Reading Food Labels

Always check ingredient labels every time you buy a packaged product. Manufacturers will frequently change the recipe, the manufacturing process, or the vendors who supply ingredients. Sometimes an allergen may be introduced with each subsequent change. If you are unsure of the product's "safeness," contact the manufacturer to ask.

The Food Allergy Labeling Consumer Protection Act of 2006 requires food manufacturers to clearly indicate the presence of the top eight allergens on food labels: peanut, tree nuts, milk, egg, fish, shellfish, wheat, and soy.

Words Indicating Gluten

Barley
Caramel color
Flour
Hydrolyzed Vegetable Protein (HVP)
Malt
Modified food starch
Monosodium Glutamate (MSG)
Oat
Rye
Spelt

Stabilizers
Starch
Sweetener
Triticale
Wheat

Foods Containing Gluten

Barley pearls	Muffins
Beers (barley)	Oatmeal
Breads and breading	Oat flour
Cake	Pasta
Cold cereals	Pretzels
Cookies	Sausages
Custard	Soft tortillas
Crackers	Soy sauce
Cream of wheat	Soups
Crusts	Starchy foods listed as "wheat-free"
Deli meat	
Distilled vinegar	
Granola bars	
Gravy	
Hot dogs	

Words Indicating Casein (Milk)

Caramel coloring
Cream
Dairy
Lactalbumin
Lactoglobulin
"Lactose-Free"
Maltodextrin
Whey

Foods Containing Casein (Milk)

Butter	Ice cream
Cheeses	Imitation cheeses
(Milk) Chocolate	"Non-dairy" creamer
Cow's milk	Puddings
Custard	Salad dressings
Deli meat	Sauces
Goat's milk (its protein is similar to cow's milk)	Sausages
	Smoothies
Hot dogs	Yogurt

Words Indicating Egg	Foods Containing Egg
Albumin	Baked goods (breads, cakes, cookies, crusts, etc.)
Dairy	
Emulsifier	Egg substitute
Globulin	Mayonnaise
Livetin	Powdered eggs
Ovomucin	Quiche
Ovomucoid	
Vitelin	

Words Indicating Soy	Foods Containing Soy
Caramel color	Chocolate candy
Emulsifier	Hot dogs
Protein	Salad dressings
Soy lecithin	Sausages
Textured Vegetable Protein (TVP)	Smooth beverages
Vegetable protein	Soy milk
	Soy sauce
	Tofu
	Vegan dishes
	"Vegetable" oil
	Vegetarian dishes

Words Indicating Peanut	Foods Containing Peanut
Green peas (direct relative of peanut)	Nuts (high chance for cross-contamination during processing)
Peanut butter	
Peanut oil	
Peanuts	
	Trail mixes
	Roasted seeds (high chance for cross-contamination during processing)

Words Indicating Tree Nuts	Foods Containing Tree Nuts
(Often cross-contaminated with peanut products and seeds)	Candy bars
	Cookies
Almonds	Flavored coffees
Brazil nuts	Nut butters
Cashews	Salads
Chestnuts	Thai dishes
Hazelnuts	Trail mixes
Macadamia nuts	
Pecans	
Pine nuts	
Pistachios	
Walnuts	

Words Indicating Rice	Foods Containing Rice
Maltodextrin	Brown rice
Starch	Corn cakes (some brands)
	Rice cakes
	Rice cereal
	Rice milk
	Starchy foods listed as "gluten-free" or "wheat-free"
	Wild rice

Words Indicating Fish/ Shellfish	Foods Containing Fish/ Shellfish
Anchovy	Asian dishes, sauces
Caviar	Cajun dishes
Crab	Imitation crabmeat
Fish	Pizza topping
Lobster	Seafood salad
Mussels	Surf and turf menus
Sardine	
Scallops	
Seafood	
Shrimp	
Tuna	

PUDDINGS

BISCUITS

SOUPS

OSTINGS

SANDY

PI

CAKE

MEAT

Main Dishes

The Autism Cookbook

1

Apple Chicken Sausage

1   LB GROUND CHICKEN (DARK MEAT)
1   MEDIUM APPLE (ANY VARIETY),
    PEELED AND FINELY CHOPPED
1   TABLESPOON GROUND SAGE
2   TEASPOONS SALT
1   TABLESPOON MOLASSES
2   TEASPOONS GROUND BLACK
    PEPPER

1. Combine all ingredients in a bowl and mix until well blended. Cover tightly and refrigerate at least 3 hours (best results if marinated overnight).

2. Use hands to form small sausage patties. Heat a frying pan to medium and cook 3–4 patties until done on each side.

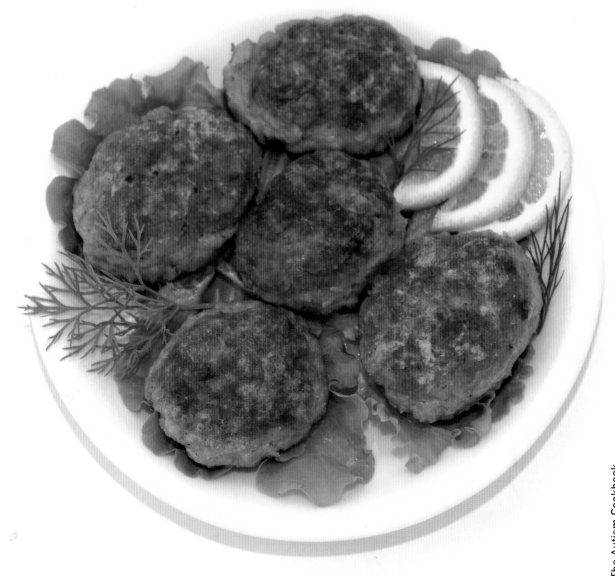

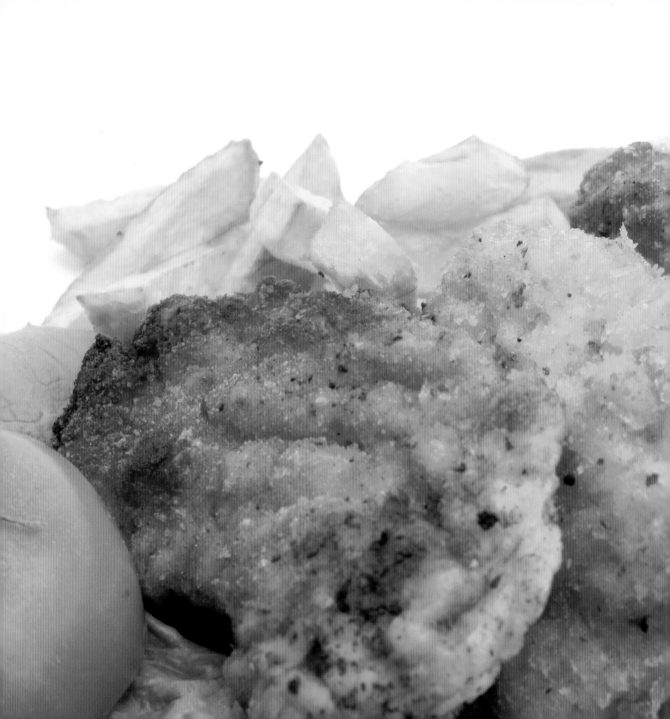

Chicken Fingers

CORN OR CANOLA OIL FOR FRYING
1   CUP CORN MEAL
2   TEASPOONS SALT
1   LARGE BONELESS, SKINLESS
    CHICKEN BREAST

1. Preheat oil in a deep fryer.

2. Line a plate with two layers of paper towels. Set aside.

3. Combine corn meal and salt in a medium bowl. Stir and set aside.

4. Wash chicken and cut into 6 to 8 slices.

5. Place chicken slices in the bowl with the corn meal. Cover chicken thoroughly with cornmeal.

6. Deep-fry approximately 2 minutes or until chicken appears light brown. Stir frequently to prevent chicken from sticking together.

7. Remove from oil. Place on the lined plate to drain excess oil.

8. Cool before serving.

Chicken Nuggets

CORN OR CANOLA OIL FOR FRYING
¼ CUP POTATO FLOUR
1½ TEASPOONS SALT
½ LB GROUND CHICKEN
¼ TEASPOON DRIED, CRUSHED THYME
    LEAVES
½ TEASPOON BLACK PEPPER

1. Preheat oil in a deep fryer.

2. Line a plate with two layers of paper towels. Set aside.

3. Combine potato flour and salt in a small bowl. Stir and set aside.

4. Combine chicken, thyme, and black pepper in a medium bowl. Stir with a fork until chicken is smooth.

5. Add flour mixture to chicken. Blend thoroughly with a fork until smooth.

6. Use hands to form half dollar–sized nuggets.

7. Stir frequently to distribute heat evenly.

8. Deep fry until medium-brown (approximately 60 – 90 seconds). Do not over-cook; potato flour burns quickly.

9. Remove nuggets from deep fryer and drain excess oil on a lined plate.

10. Cool before serving.

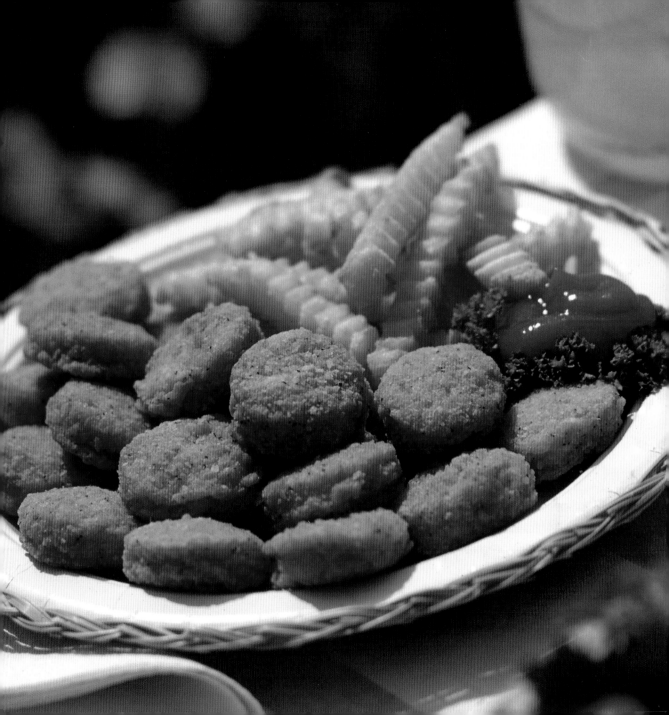

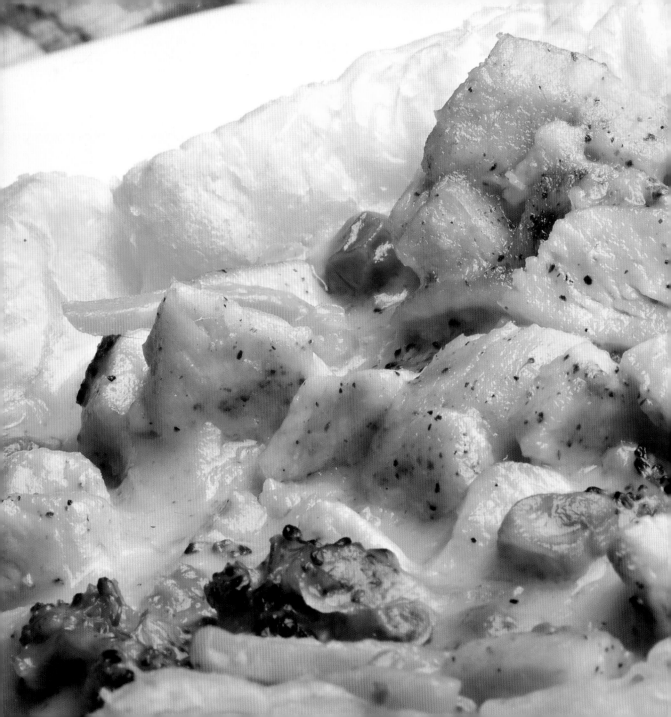

Chicken Potpie

CRUMB TOPPING
¼ CUP CORN OR CANOLA OIL OR ¼ CUP PALM OIL SHORTENING
1 TEASPOON SALT
2 CUPS QUINOA FLOUR OR BUCKWHEAT FLOUR
½ CUP COLD WATER

FILLING
1 TABLESPOON OLIVE OIL
½ LB BONELESS, SKINLESS CHICKEN BREASTS CUT INTO CUBES
4 CUPS CHICKEN BROTH
1 TEASPOON SALT
1 TEASPOON GROUND BLACK PEPPER
1 CUP EACH OF CHOPPED CARROTS, BROCOLLI, AND CUT STRING BEANS
1 SMALL ONION, CHOPPED
1 LARGE RUSSET POTATO, PEELED AND CHOPPED
2 CUPS WATER
2 TABLESPOONS POTATO FLOUR

1. Prepare topping: Combine oil (or shortening), salt, and flour in a small bowl. Stir with a fork until blended. Add 1 tablespoon of water and stir. Keep adding 1 tablespoon and stirring until flour mixture is crumbly and not too wet. Set aside.

2. Prepare filling: Heat olive oil to low setting in a medium-sized pot. Cook chicken 3–4 minutes on all sides.

3. Add chicken broth, salt, pepper, carrots, string beans, broccoli, onions, and potatoes. Bring to a boil. Reduce heat and simmer on low for 15 minutes.

4. Meanwhile, whisk potato flour and water in a small cup until potato flour is dissolved. Slowly pour into the chicken broth pot while stirring. Boil and stir an additional 2 minutes on low. Mixture will thicken.

5. Pour all ingredients into a casserole dish. Sprinkle topping evenly over filling. Bake at 400°F for approximately 30 minutes or until topping appears light brown and the filling bubbles over the edges of the topping.

Chicken-Sausage Ratatouille

¼ CUP OLIVE OIL

2 BONELESS, SKINLESS CHICKEN BREASTS, CUBED

2 CUPS OF SMOKED SAUSAGE OR KIELBASA, SLICED

4 GARLIC CLOVES, MINCED

1 CUP ZUCCHINI SQUASH, CUBED

1 CUP EGGPLANT, PEELED AND CUBED

1 CUP RED BELL PEPPER, CHOPPED

1 CUP WATER

2 CUPS TOMATO, CUBED

1 TABLESPOON DRIED, CRUSHED OREGANO

5 FRESH BASIL LEAVES, CHOPPED

1. In a small Dutch oven, combine oil and meat. Cook over medium temperature until chicken is slightly brown, stirring constantly.

2. Stir in garlic, zucchini, eggplant, and bell pepper. Cook until zucchini is slightly soft.

3. Stir in water, tomato, oregano, and basil. The mixture should be very thick.

4. Cover tightly and let simmer on low temperature for 25–30 minutes. Stir occasionally to prevent sticking to the bottom.

5. Cool slightly and serve.

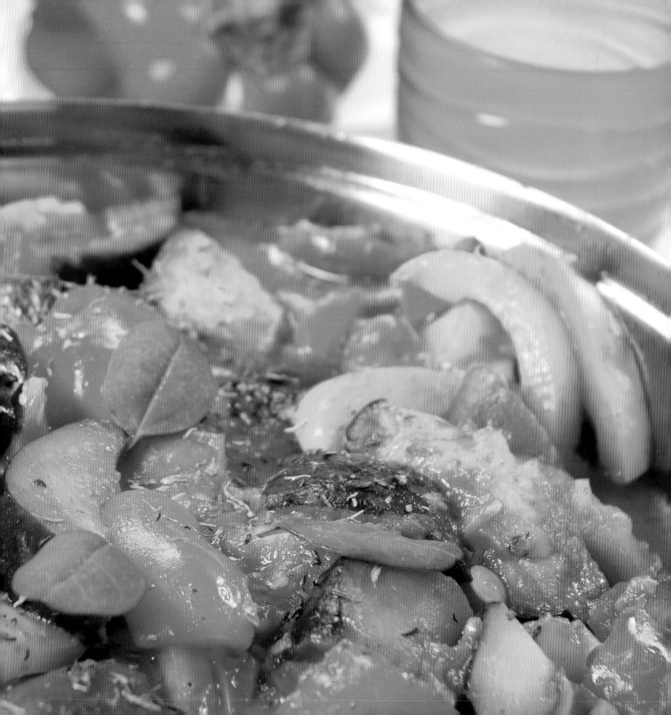

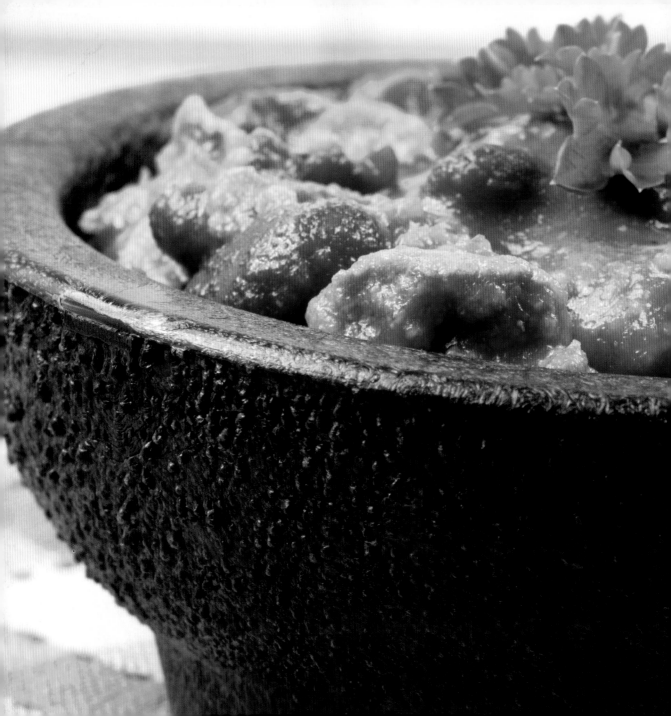

Chunky Red Bean Chili

½ LB GROUND TURKEY OR GROUND CHUCK BEEF
½ CUP EXTRA VIRGIN OLIVE OIL
1 SMALL GREEN PEPPER, CHOPPED
½ CUP ONION, CHOPPED
2 GARLIC CLOVES, MINCED
2 TABLESPOONS GROUND CUMIN
½ TEASPOON BLACK PEPPER
½ TEASPOON SALT
1 CAN (14–16 OUNCES) RED BEANS, DRAINED (DO NOT RINSE)
2 CUPS TOMATO SAUCE
½ CUP FRESH CILANTRO LEAVES, CHOPPED

1. In a medium pot, brown the meat. Drain any excess fat.

2. Add olive oil, green pepper, onion, garlic, cumin, black pepper, and salt. Simmer over low heat until vegetables are soft. Stir occasionally.

3. Add drained beans and tomato sauce. Stir until blended.

4. Simmer over very low heat approximately 1 hour, stirring occasionally.

5. Add cilantro. Stir and continue to simmer over very low heat for an additional 30 minutes. Chili will thicken.

Chunky Vegetable Chili (Raw)

1 PORTOBELLO MUSHROOM, CUBED
1 MEDIUM ZUCCHINI, CUBED
1 LARGE TOMATO, CUBED
1 SMALL ONION, CHOPPED
2 TEASPOONS SALT
2 TABLESPOONS CUMIN POWDER
3 TABLESPOONS COLD-PRESSED
  OLIVE OIL
JUICE OF 1 LARGE LEMON

SAUCE
2 LARGE TOMATOES, CUBED
4 SUNDRIED TOMATOES
1 GARLIC CLOVE
1 CUP FRESH CILANTRO LEAVES
2 TABLESPOONS GROUND CUMIN
½ TEASPOON SALT
2 TABLESPOONS OLIVE OIL
1 CUP WATER

1. Combine chili ingredients in a large bowl. Stir until well blended.

2. Cover tightly and let marinate 30 minutes at room temperature.

3. Prepare sauce: Combine all sauce ingredients in a blender. Blend until smooth.

4. Add sauce to chili ingredients and stir until well blended.

5. Cover tightly and let marinate at room temperature for 1 hour.

6. If desired, warm slightly to no more than 118°F.

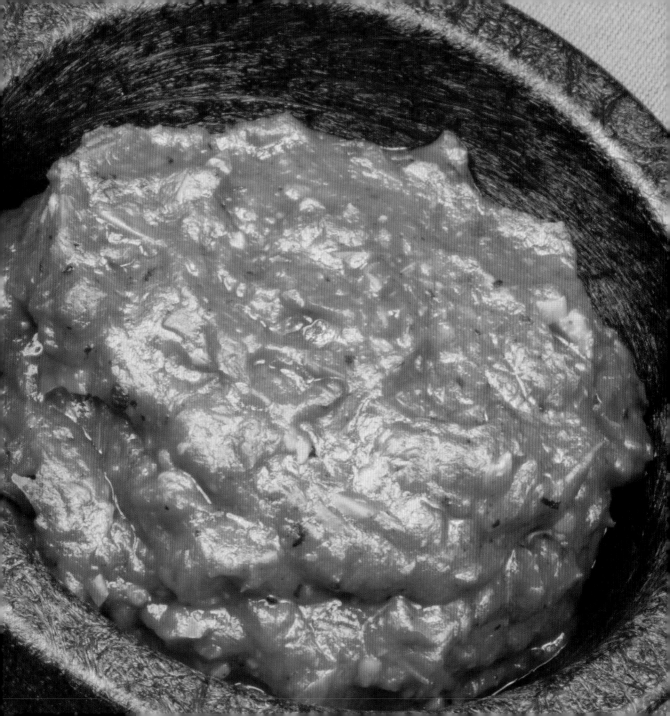

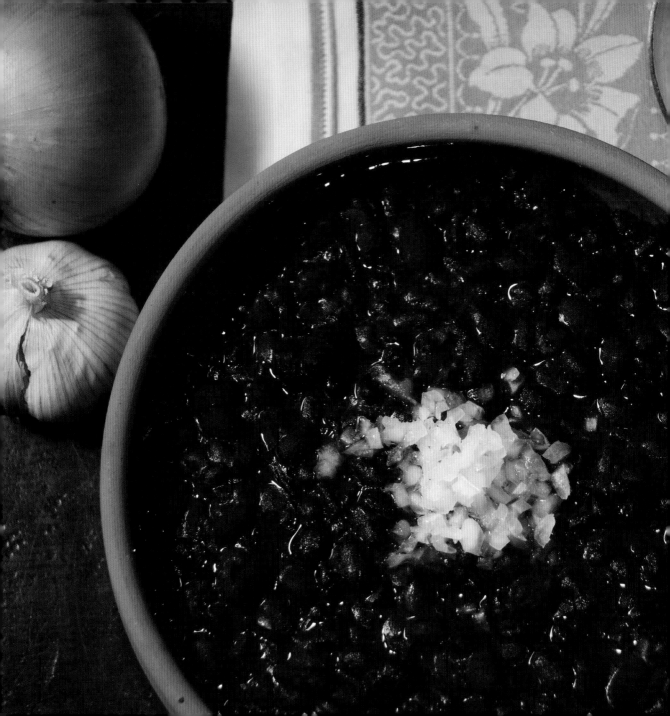

Cuban Black Beans

¼ CUP EXTRA VIRGIN OLIVE OIL
½ GREEN PEPPER, CHOPPED
1 SMALL ONION, CHOPPED
3 GARLIC CLOVES, CHOPPED
½ TEASPOON GROUND CUMIN
½ TEASPOON BLACK PEPPER
1 CAN (14–16 OUNCES) UNSEASONED
    BLACK BEANS—DO NOT DRAIN OR
    RINSE
½ LB COOKED MEAT, SUCH AS SMOKED
    TURKEY OR ROASTED PORK, IF
    DESIRED

1. Combine olive oil, green pepper, onion, garlic, cumin, and black pepper in a small saucepan. Stir while simmering on low until vegetables are soft.

2. Add black beans (with sauce). Stir until well blended.

3. Simmer over very low heat; add cooked meat for flavor if desired. Cook for 45 minutes. Stir occasionally.

Serve warm over a baked potato or over Steamed Quinoa or Buckwheat with Veggies on page 106.

Easy Chicken Quinoa Casserole

1 LARGE CHICKEN BREAST
1 CUP UNCOOKED QUINOA SEEDS
2 CUPS CHICKEN BROTH
2 TABLESPOONS OLIVE OIL
1 SMALL ONION, MINCED
1 CELERY STALK, CHOPPED
1 RED BELL PEPPER, SLICED INTO CIRCLES

1. Slice chicken breasts along the middle to make two thinner slices. Place in a bowl and season as desired. If your chicken broth contains salt, you may want to omit salt from the seasoning. Set aside.

2. Pour quinoa seeds into a 9-inch baking dish. Add broth, oil, onion, and celery and stir until quinoa is submerged.

3. Top with chicken breasts and bell peppers.

4. Cover tightly and bake 30-40 minutes until all broth is absorbed into the quinoa seeds.

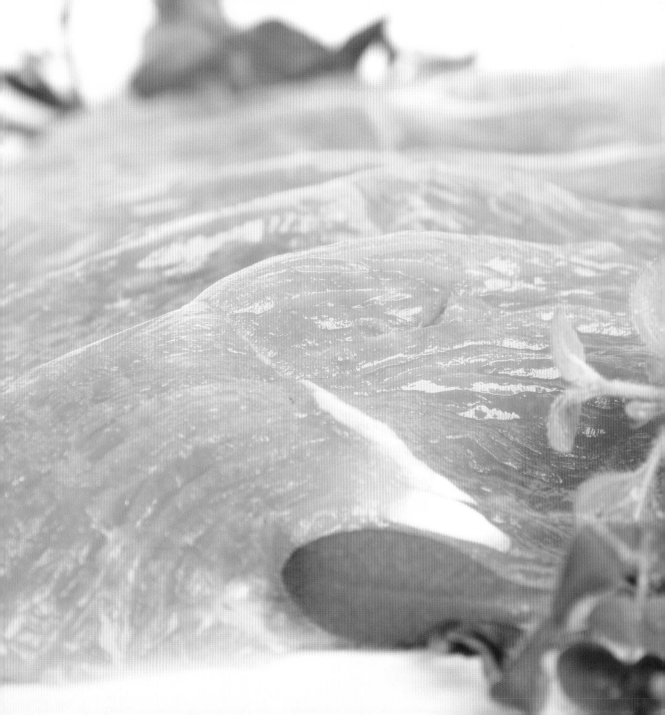

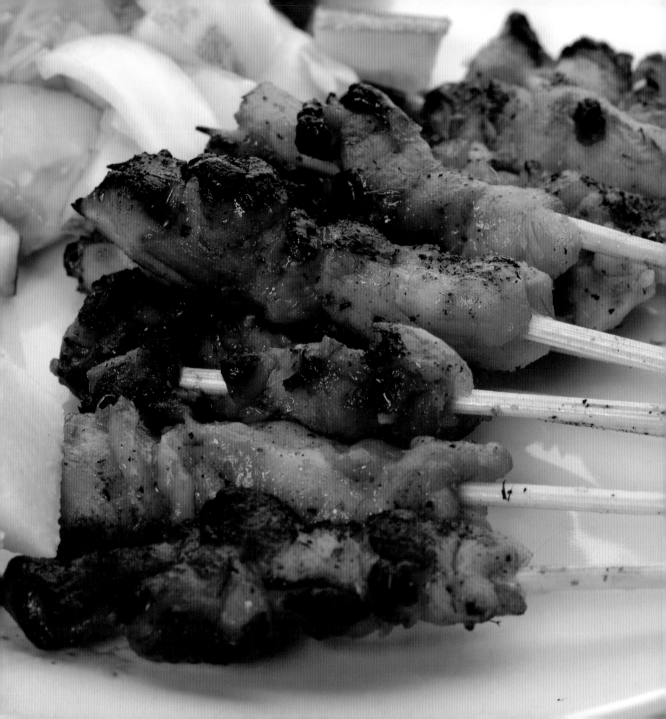

Grilled Chicken Skewers

5   BONELESS, SKINLESS CHICKEN THIGHS

¼   CUP ROASTED SESAME OIL

SWEETENER—2 TABLESPOONS EVAPORATED CANE JUICE OR ½ CUP AGAVE NECTAR

1½ TEASPOONS SALT

2   TABLESPOONS GROUND GINGER POWDER

2   GARLIC CLOVES, MINCED

1. Wash and trim excess fat from chicken thighs.

2. Cut chicken into 2-inch slices.

3. Combine chicken slices and all ingredients in a medium bowl. Stir until well blended.

4. Cover and refrigerate. Let marinate at least 20 minutes.

5. Place chicken slices on individual skewers.

6. Place skewers on grill over medium heat. Cook thoroughly on each side until done.

Dip in warm Sesame or Pumpkin "Butter" as a dip on page 221 or serve with Steamed Quinoa or Buckwheat with Veggies on page 106.

Hamburger Pie

½ LB GROUND BEEF OR TURKEY
1 SMALL ONION, CHOPPED
1 TEASPOON EACH OF SALT, BLACK
  PEPPER, AND GARLIC POWDER
½ TEASPOON CRUSHED THYME
½ CUP EACH OF FROZEN CORN AND
  SLICED CARROTS
¼ CUP TOMATO SAUCE
¼ CUP WATER
½ BATCH OF CORNBREAD (RECIPE
  FROM PAGE 129)

1. Combine meat and onion in a large pan. Cook meat until brown.

2. Add salt, pepper, garlic powder, thyme, and vegetables. Stir until blended and vegetables are thawed.

3. Stir in tomato sauce and water. Pour all ingredients into a 9-inch round pie pan. Pour cornbread batter over top of the meat. Be sure to fill in the corners of the pan with batter. If needed, use a rubber spatula to spread the batter.

4. Bake for 25–30 minutes until cornbread appears light brown and crusty.

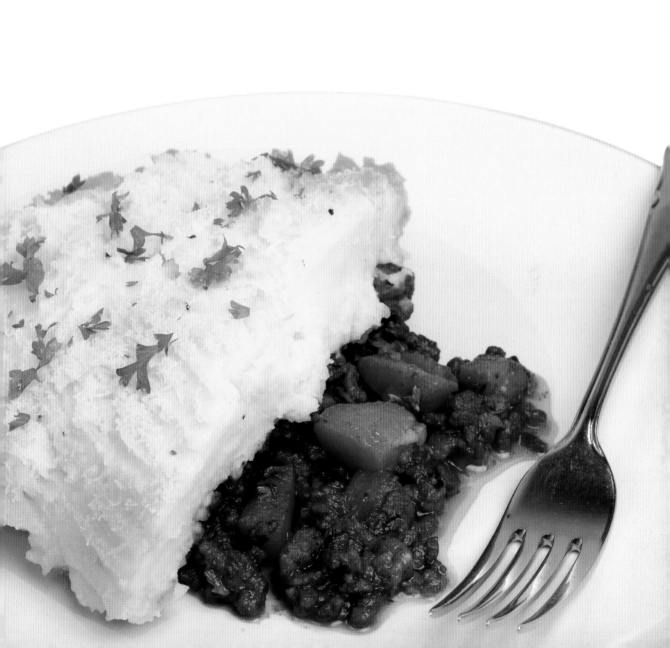

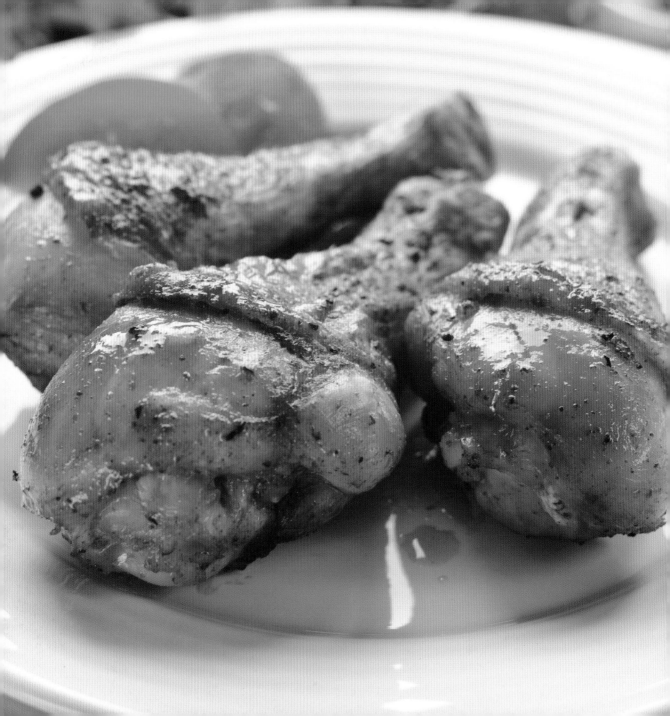

Maple-Glazed Chicken Legs

6 MEDIUM CHICKEN LEGS
1   CUP 100% MAPLE SYRUP
2   TABLESPOONS RAW APPLE CIDER
    VINEGAR
1   TEASPOON OLIVE OIL
½   TEASPOON SALT
1   TEASPOON CURRY SEASONING
    (OPTIONAL)

1. In a small mixing bowl, combine all ingredients except for chicken. Stir with a whisk until blended. In a large freezer storage bag, combine glaze ingredients and chicken legs. Seal the bag and use your hands to gently blend the maple seasoning into the chicken from the outside of the bag. Refrigerate for 1 hour. Place chicken on a glass baking dish and bake 45 minutes or until light brown.

Meatballs with Sweet Glaze

½ LB GROUND BEEF OR TURKEY
2 CUPS ITALIAN-STYLE
   BREADCRUMBS ON PAGE 134
½ CUP TOMATO SAUCE
2 TABLESPOONS EXTRA VIRGIN OLIVE
   OIL

GLAZE
2 CUPS TOMATO SAUCE
2 CUPS FRESH CRANBERRIES
1 CUP AGAVE NECTAR OR
   EVAPORATED CANE JUICE

1. In a medium mixing bowl, combine turkey, breadcrumbs, and tomato sauce. Mix with a large spoon until smooth. Use your hands to form 1-inch balls. In a large saucepan, heat olive oil at a low setting. Cook meatballs thoroughly on each side.

2. Prepare glaze: Combine tomato sauce, cranberries, and sweetener in a small pot. Heat over a low setting for 10 minutes. Stir frequently until cranberries are limp. Pour glaze over meatballs, with or without the cranberry chunks.

3. Cool slightly before serving.

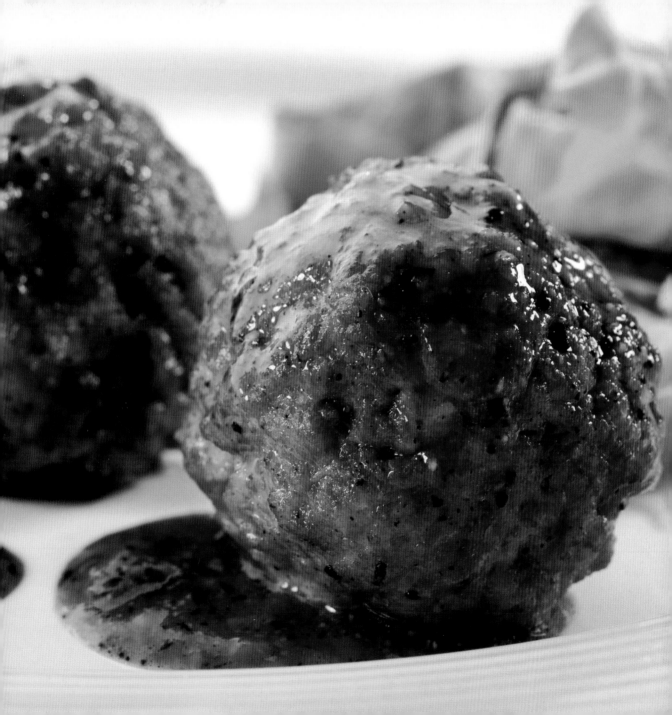

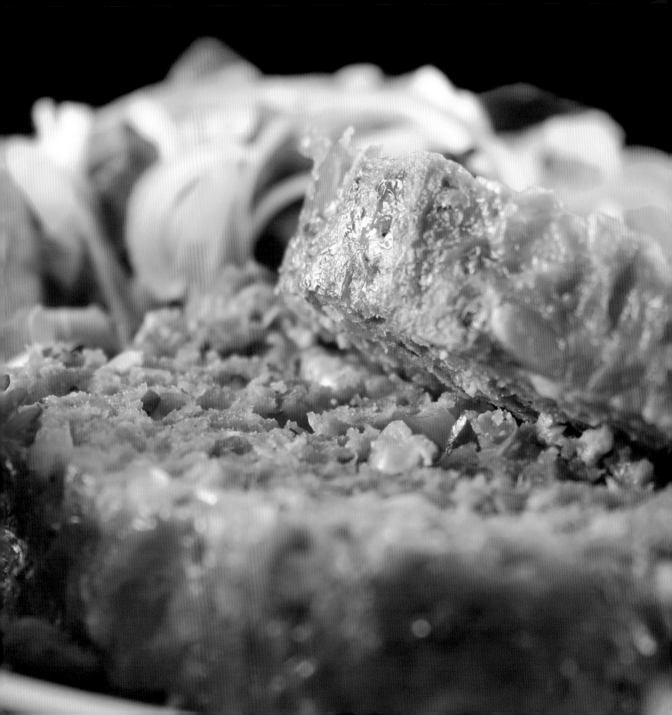

Meatloaf

1½ LBS LEAN GROUND BEEF OR
    TURKEY
1   SMALL ONION, FINELY CHOPPED
½   SMALL GREEN PEPPER, FINELY
    CHOPPED
1½ CUPS BREADCRUMBS ON PAGE 134
    OR ½ CUP BUCKWHEAT FLOUR
4   TABLESPOONS EXTRA VIRGIN OLIVE
    OIL
1½ CUPS TOMATO SAUCE
1   TABLESPOON DRIED, CRUSHED
    OREGANO LEAVES
2   TABLESPOONS GARLIC POWDER
1   TEASPOON BLACK PEPPER
1   TEASPOON SALT (OPTIONAL)

TOPPINGS
½   CUP TOMATO SAUCE OR KETCHUP
1   TEASPOON DRIED, CRUSHED
    OREGANO LEAVES

1. Preheat oven to 400°F.

2. Combine all meatloaf ingredients in a large mixing bowl. Mix well with a large fork until the mixture is smooth.

3. Spread meat evenly into a 9 x 5-inch loaf pan.

4. Smooth tomato sauce or ketchup over top. Sprinkle lightly with oregano.

5. Bake on middle rack of oven until sides of meatloaf are slightly brown and crusty (approximately 45 minutes).

6. Remove from pan to a serving dish.

Serve with Fluffy Mashed Potatoes on page 80.

Pasta with Creamy Sauce

TO MAKE CREAM SAUCE:

3   CUPS CHICKEN BROTH
½   CUP OLIVE OIL
¼   CUP BUCKWHEAT FLOUR
3   CUPS CHICKEN BROTH
½   TEASPOON GARLIC POWDER
1   TEASPOON FINELY CRUSHED THYME
     LEAVES
1   TEASPOON SALT

1. Prepare gluten-free pasta of your choice. Drain, rinse, and set aside.

1. In a medium saucepan, combine oil and broth. Stir over medium heat until the mixture is smooth. Add flour, garlic powder, thyme, and salt. Stir with a whisk until smooth. Simmer over low heat for 3 minutes. Serve warm over pasta.

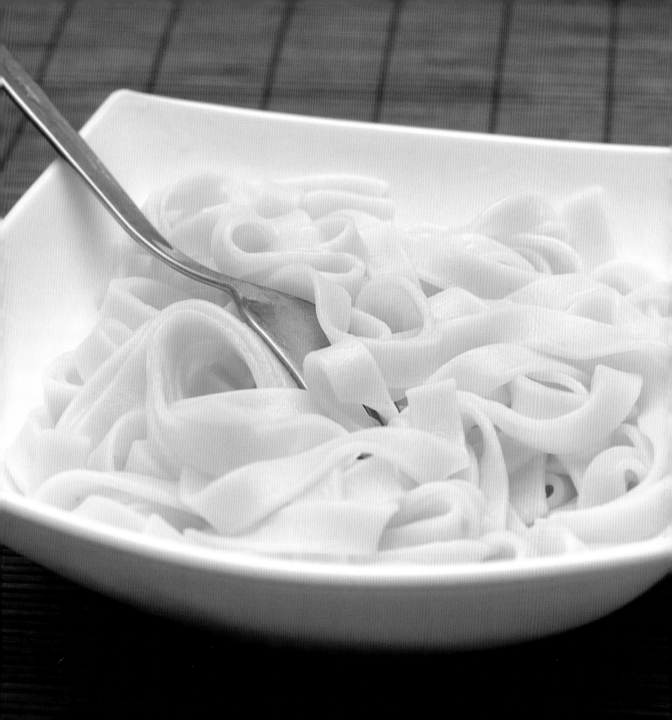

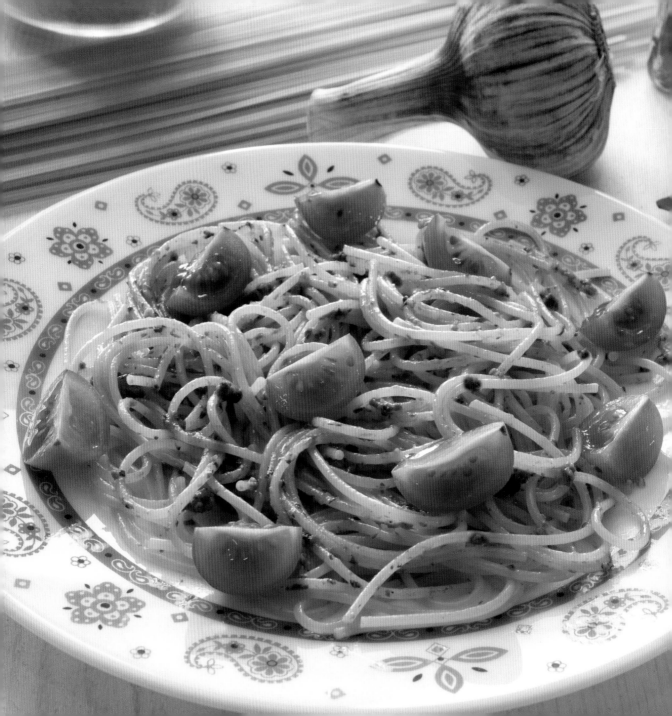

Pasta with Garlic Sauce

1 CUP CORN OR CANOLA OIL
5 GARLIC CLOVES, MINCED
1 TEASPOON SALT
2 TEASPOONS GROUND BLACK
  PEPPER
3 STRIPS OF UNCURED TURKEY
  BACON, COOKED AND CHOPPED
2 MEDIUM MUSHROOMS, SLICED
3 CHERRY TOMATOES, SLICED IN HALF
3 FRESH BASIL LEAVES, CHOPPED
½ LB COOKED CORN SPAGHETTI

1. In a small saucepan, combine oil, garlic, salt, and black pepper. Simmer over very low heat until garlic is brown.

2. Add bacon, mushrooms, tomato, and basil. Continue to simmer and stir over very low heat for 3 minutes. Stir frequently.

3. Remove from heat and pour over hot, cooked corn or quinoa pasta. Toss vigorously to distribute sauce.

Serve warm. If desired, add cooked slices of chicken breast.

Pizza

1 CUP BUCKWHEAT FLOUR
½ TEASPOON SALT
1 TEASPOON ALUMINUM-FREE
  BAKING POWDER
2 TABLESPOONS PALM OIL
  SHORTENING
UP TO ½ CUP COLD WATER

SUGGESTED TOPPINGS
  GARLIC POWDER
  CRUSHED OREGANO LEAVES
  TOMATO SAUCE
  COOKED ITALIAN SAUSAGE AND/OR
    GROUND TURKEY
  GREEN PEPPERS

1. Preheat oven to 375°F.

2. In a large bowl combine flour, salt, and baking powder. Sift with a fork.

3. Add shortening and ¼ cup of water. Stir until blended. Add more water until dough sticks together.

4. Use your hands to form a ball. If necessary, dust very lightly with flour to prevent sticking. Knead the dough for 1 minute.

5. Place dough on a pizza pan or cookie sheet. Use your hands to form a flat 8-inch crust. Lift the ends slightly to form an outer crust.

6. Sprinkle garlic powder and oregano over the surface. Spread tomato sauce and other desired toppings.

7. If desired, combine olive oil and cornmeal in a small bowl. Brush lightly onto outer crust.

8. Bake on the middle rack of the oven for approximately 30–45 minutes or until outer crust is light brown.

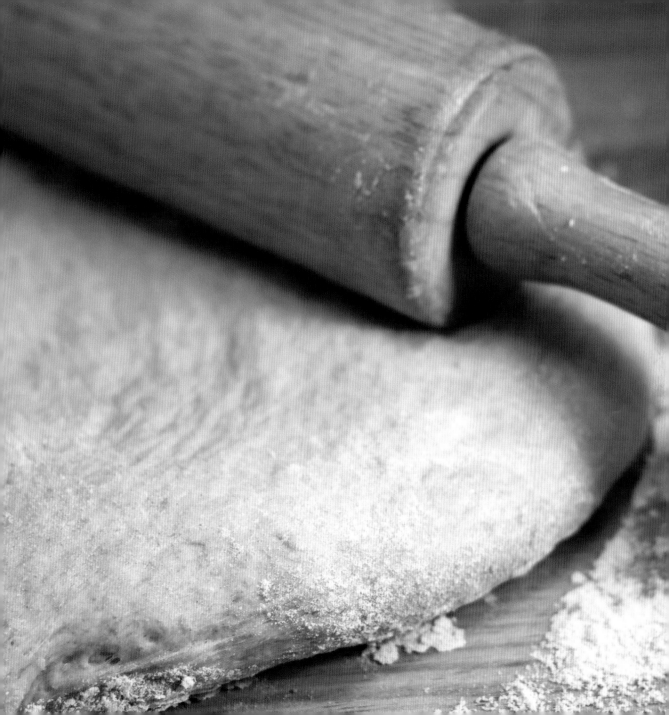

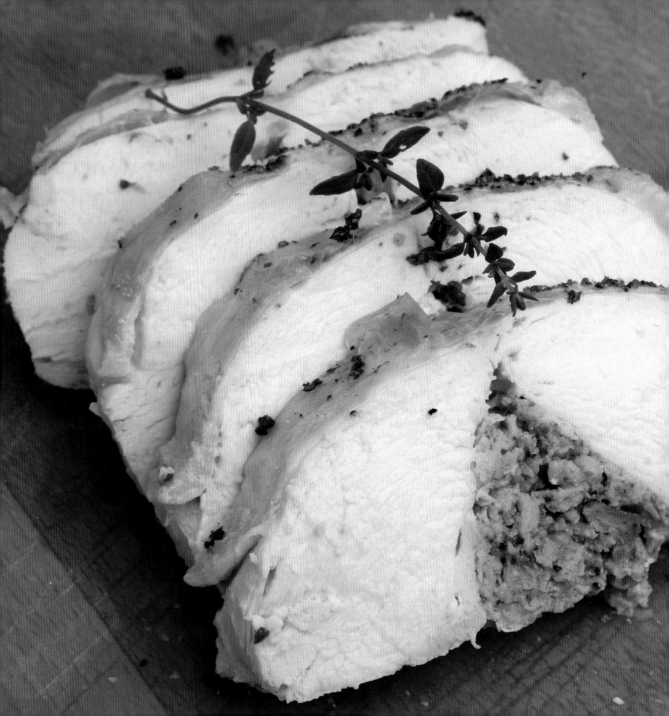

Pumpkin Seed & Apple Stuffed Chicken

1 TABLESPOON CORN OR CANOLA OIL FOR SAUTÉING

1 TEASPOON EACH OF SALT AND GROUND BLACK PEPPER

¼ CUP ONION, FINELY CHOPPED

½ CUP ROASTED PUMPKIN SEEDS, FINELY CHOPPED IN FOOD PROCESSOR

1 TABLESPOON FLAX SEED MEAL

½ CUP CORNMEAL

¼ CUP OF APPLE, PEELED AND FINELY CHOPPED

½ TEASPOON EACH OF GROUND CINNAMON, CARDAMOM (OPTIONAL), AND NUTMEG

½ CUP WATER

2 LARGE BONELESS, SKINLESS CHICKEN BREASTS, SLICED HORIZONTALLY TO SPREAD OPEN

1. Pour oil, salt, pepper, and onion into a small skillet and cook the onion until soft. In a medium mixing bowl, combine cooked onion and all other ingredients. Stir until well blended. The stuffing should be very thick.

2. Cut open the chicken breasts to lay flat. Scoop 2–3 tablespoons of stuffing mix and spread onto one side of the chicken. Fold the chicken to close. Place stuffed chicken on baking dish two inches apart. Brush lightly with oil. Bake uncovered for 45 minutes. Cool slightly. Slice and serve.

Quick Stew

5 BONELESS, SKINLESS CHICKEN
 THIGHS OR 1 LB SIRLOIN BEEF
 CUBES
¼ CUP EXTRA VIRGIN OLIVE OIL
3 CUPS FRESH TOMATO, CUBED
1 MEDIUM ONION, SLICED
2 TEASPOONS EACH OF DRIED,
 CRUSHED BASIL, OREGANO, AND
 THYME LEAVES
2 CUPS WATER
½ CUP POTATO, PEELED AND CUBED
SALT AND PEPPER TO TASTE
4 GARLIC CLOVES, MINCED

1. Use a large saucepan to heat olive oil over medium heat. Add chicken or beef and brown lightly on all sides.

2. Add tomatoes, onion, basil, oregano, thyme, salt, and pepper.

3. Set temperature to low. Add water and potato and cover tightly.

4. Simmer 30 minutes for chicken and 60 minutes for beef.

5. Open lid and sprinkle garlic over top of the meat. Do not stir.

6. Cover tightly again. Simmer on low for an additional 15 minutes.

Serve over steamed quinoa.

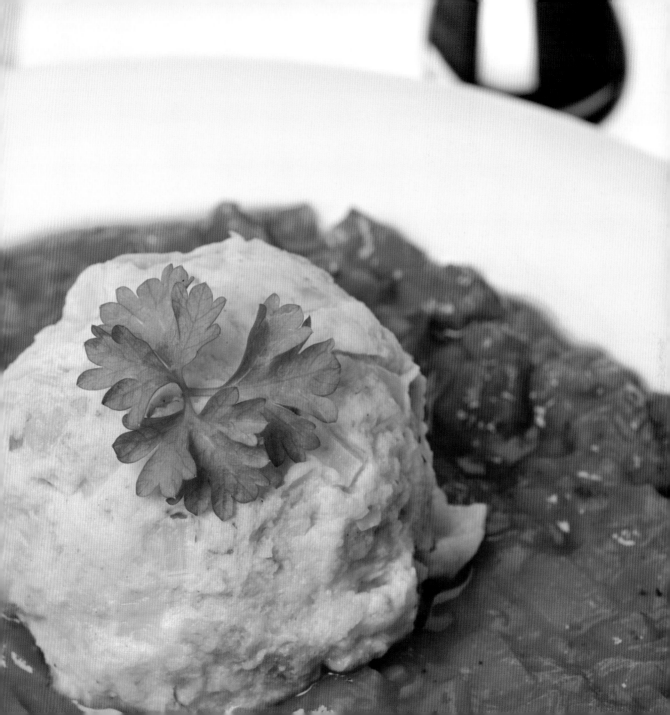

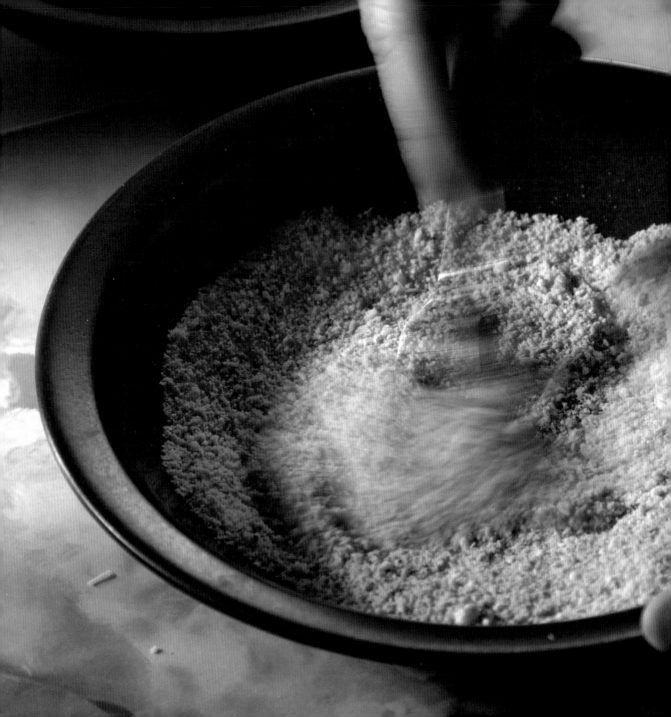

Seed-Crusted Chicken Breast

2   TABLESPOONS OLIVE OIL
½   TEASPOON SALT
2   BONELESS, SKINLESS CHICKEN
    BREASTS

CRUSTING
½   CUP PUMPKIN SEEDS (LIGHTLY
    ROASTED WITHOUT OIL)
1   TABLESPOON FLAX SEED MEAL
    (OPTIONAL)
½   TEASPOON GROUND CUMIN
½   TEASPOON GROUND CORIANDER
1   TEASPOON GROUND BLACK PEPPER

1. Season chicken breasts in oil and salt. Set aside in the refrigerator for at least one hour.

2. Preheat oven to 400°F. Combine all crusting ingredients in a blender. Blend on high speed until ingredients are flaky. Pour into a medium bowl. Dip chicken into crusting, covering each side completely. Place chicken on oiled baking dish and bake uncovered for 45–60 minutes or until chicken appears light brown.

Sesame-Ginger Chicken

5   BONELESS, SKINLESS CHICKEN
    THIGHS
½   CUP ROASTED SESAME OIL
3   TABLESPOONS FRESH GINGER,
    PEELED AND FINELY CHOPPED
2   TEASPOONS SALT
1   TEASPOON BLACK PEPPER
1   CUP WATER
5   GARLIC CLOVES, MINCED
½   GREEN PEPPER, CHOPPED
3   WHOLE SCALLIONS, SLICED
¼   CUP ROASTED SESAME SEEDS

1. Wash chicken thoroughly and drain excess water.

2. Remove excess fat with a knife and discard.

3. Combine meat, sesame oil, ginger, salt, and black pepper in a large bowl. Mix thoroughly.

4. Brown the chicken on each side in a hot skillet (do not use additional oil).

5. Reduce temperature to medium-low. Add water and cover tightly. Simmer 30 minutes or until chicken is tender.

6. Scatter garlic, green pepper, scallions, and sesame seeds over top of the meat. Do not stir.

7. Cover tightly again and simmer on low for an additional 15 minutes.

    Serve with a baked potato or with Asian Noodles on page 65. Also great with Steamed Quinoa or Buckwheat with Veggies on page 106.

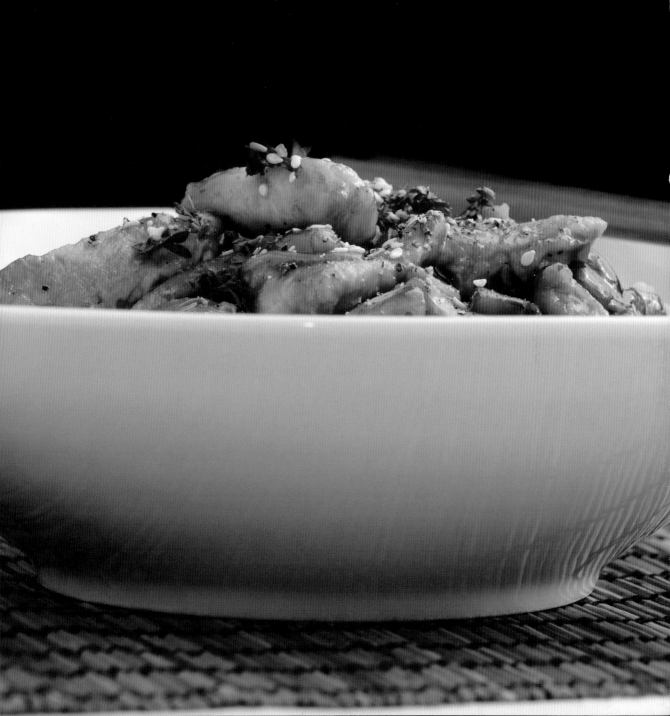

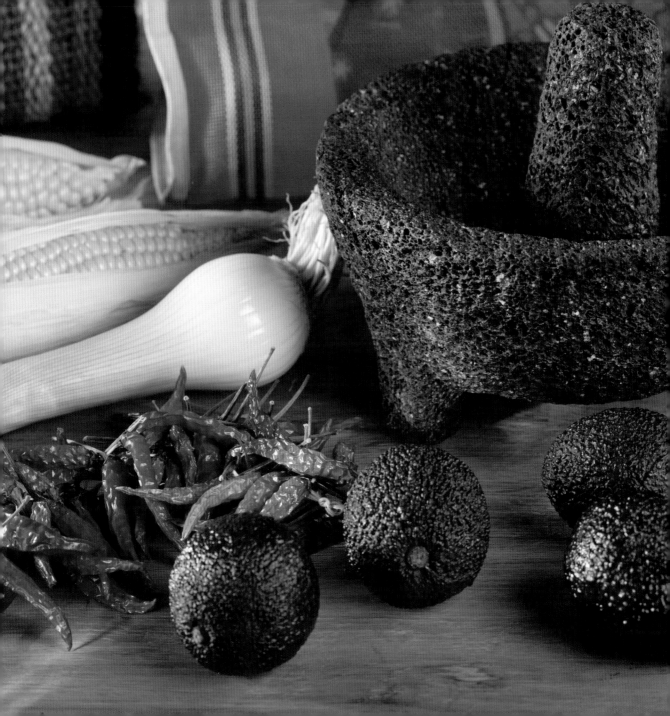

Shredded Chicken Enchiladas

6 SOFT ALL-CORN TORTILLAS
  (AVAILABLE IN THE BREAD AISLE OF
  MOST GROCERY STORES)

SAUCE:
2 CUPS TOMATO SAUCE
2 TABLESPOONS GROUND CUMIN
  POWDER
2 TABLESPOONS GARLIC POWDER
1 TEASPOON SALT
½ TEASPOON GROUND BLACK PEPPER
1 TEASPOON BUCKWHEAT FLOUR
  (OPTIONAL—AS A THICKENER)

FILLING:
3 TABLESPOONS OLIVE OIL
1 SMALL ONION, PEELED AND SLICED
1 SMALL GREEN BELL PEPPER,
  PEELED AND SLICED
2 LARGE BONELESS, SKINLESS
  CHICKEN BREASTS, SLICED
  THROUGH THE MIDDLE TO MAKE 4
  THIN PIECES

1. Prepare sauce: Combine tomato sauce, cumin, garlic powder, salt, and black pepper in a medium pot. Bring to a simmer over low heat. While stirring, slowly add the buckwheat flour. Continue to stir until sauce thickens. Remove from heat and set aside.

2. Prepare Filling: In a large frying pan, heat olive oil and add chicken, cilantro, onion, and green pepper. Cook chicken thoroughly on each side and stir vegetables until soft. Remove from heat. Pour in ½ of the sauce. Use a fork and knife to shred the chicken. Spoon the mixture into the center of the corn tortillas. Gently fold to close and place enchiladas in a baking dish, side by side. Pour remaining sauce over the enchiladas. Bake uncovered for 15–20 minutes.

Slow Cooker Barbecue Chicken

2   BONELESS, SKINLESS CHICKEN
    BREASTS
2   CUPS BARBECUE SAUCE (FROM
    RECIPE ON PAGE 219)
½   CUP OF WATER
4   SLICES OF GREEN PEPPER

1. Place chicken, barbecue sauce, and water in a slow
    cooker. Stir until blended. Place green pepper slices
    on top. Set temperature to medium heat. Cover and
    cook for 6–7 hours. Shred the chicken and wrap in
    a soft corn tortilla or serve with salad greens and a
    corn muffin.

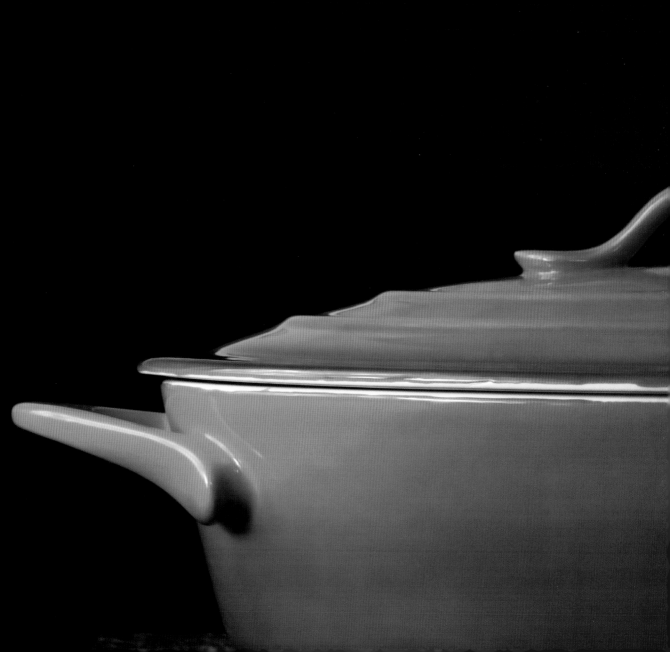

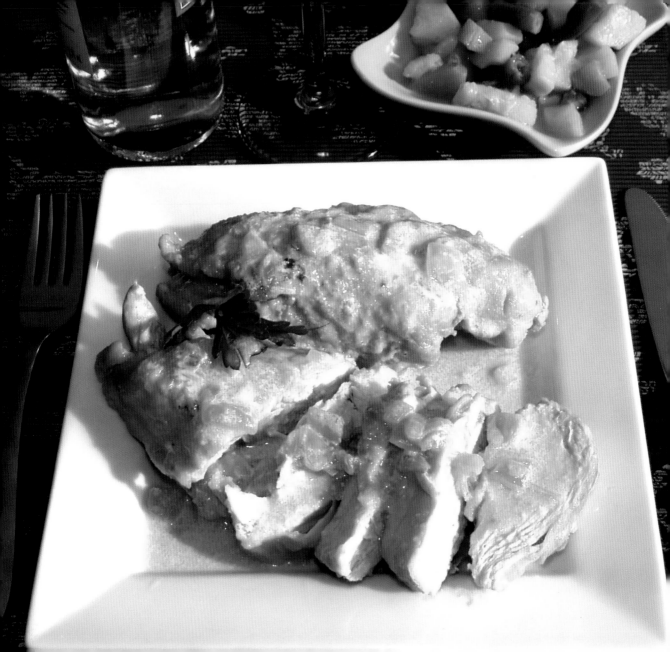

Smothered Chicken

1 TABLESPOON OLIVE OIL
½ RED ONION, SLICED
1 RED BELL PEPPER, SLICED
½ TEASPOON SALT
½ TEASPOON GROUND BLACK PEPPER
½ TEASPOON GARLIC POWDER
4 BONELESS, SKINLESS CHICKEN
   BREASTS

GRAVY
3 CUPS OF WATER
¼ CUP POTATO FLOUR

1. Heat olive oil on low in a large skillet. Cook chicken until brown on each side. Add onions, bell peppers, salt, black pepper, and garlic powder. Cook until the onions are slightly brown. Cover and let simmer on lowest setting.

2. Prepare gravy: Combine potato flour and water in a large cup. Whisk until the flour is dissolved.

3. Pour potato flour mixture over chicken and bring to a simmer.

4. Reduce heat to low. Simmer for 20–30 minutes or until chicken is tender. Stir frequently.

Stuffed Peppers

4 MEDIUM BELL PEPPERS, HOLLOWED (ANY COLOR)
½ LB GROUND BEEF OR TURKEY
2 CUPS TOMATO SAUCE
4 GARLIC CLOVES, MINCED
1 SMALL ONION, FINELY CHOPPED
2 TEASPOONS SALT
2 TEASPOONS CRUSHED OREGANO LEAVES
½ CUP UNCOOKED BUCKWHEAT SEEDS

1. Preheat oven to 350°F.

2. Brown the meat in a medium sauce pan. Add tomato sauce, garlic, and seasonings. Simmer on low for 5 minutes. Pour ingredients into a large mixing bowl and add buckwheat seeds. Stir until well blended. Spoon the mixture into peppers until full.

3. Place peppers upright on a baking sheet and bake for 30 minutes or until edges of the peppers are lightly browned. Cool slightly before serving.

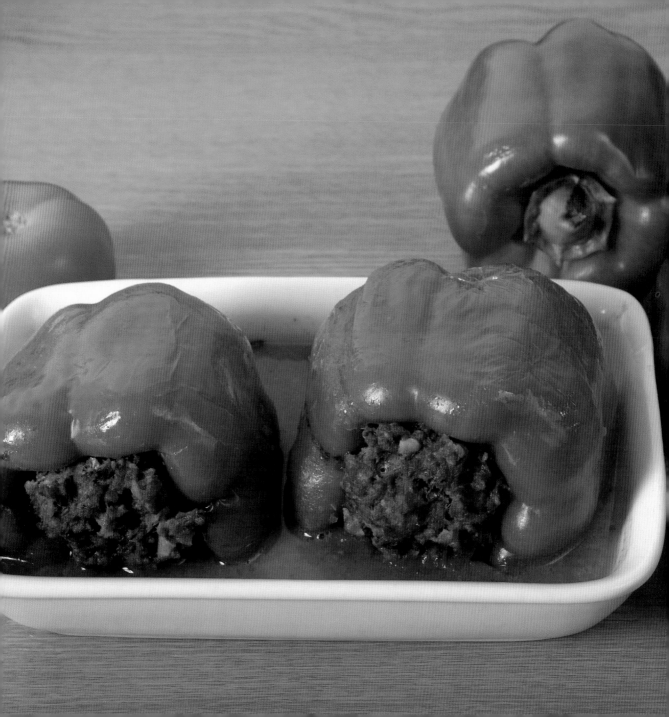

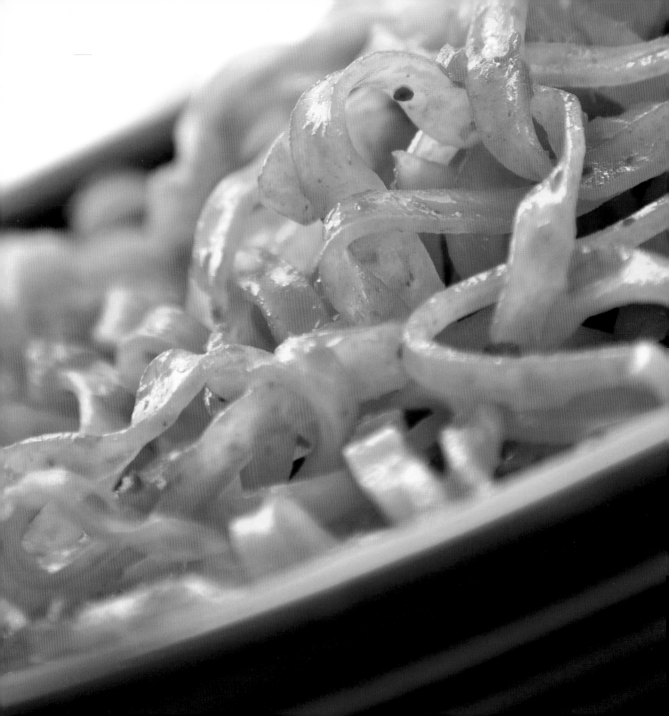

Thai Noodles with Sesame Butter Sauce

12 OUNCES OF UNCOOKED SPAGHETTI
OR LINGUINI PASTA (CORN OR
QUINOA VARIETIES)
2 TABLESPOONS OLIVE OIL
SESAME BUTTER (FROM PAGE 221)
¼ CUP COCONUT MILK
2 TABLESPOONS CURRY POWDER
1 TABLESPOON CUMIN POWDER
CRUSHED THYME (GARNISH)

1. Cook the pasta. Rinse and drain. Pour in 2 tablespoons of olive oil and toss. Set aside. Prepare Sesame Butter recipe and add coconut milk, curry powder, and cumin powder while blending. Pour sesame butter mixture over pasta and toss. Drizzle more sesame butter on top and garnish with crushed thyme. Serve warm.

Add slices of grilled chicken if desired.

Turkey or Beef Turnovers

PASTRY:
2 CUPS BUCKWHEAT FLOUR
1 TEASPOON APPLE CIDER VINEGAR
1 TEASPOON OLIVE OIL
½ CUP BOILING HOT WATER
EXTRA FLOUR FOR DUSTING

1. Place flour in a medium-sized mixing bowl. Make a well in the center of the dough. Pour vinegar, oil, and hot water into the center and stir until ingredients are blended. Make a ball with your hands and knead for five minutes. Dust with extra flour if too sticky. Lightly dust the bottom of parchment paper with flour. Place the dough on the paper and roll out into a circle with a rolling pin until the dough is ¼-inch thick. Cut into 2-inch squares. Set aside.

FILLING
½ LB GROUND TURKEY OR BEEF
1 TABLESPOON CURRY POWDER
1 TABLESPOON CRUSHED THYME
    LEAVES
½ TEASPOON SALT
1 SMALL ONION, FINELY CHOPPED
¼ CUP WATER

1. Brown the meat in a medium saucepan. Add seasonings and water. Cover and simmer on low for 10 minutes. Cool completely. Spoon the meat into the center of the dough pieces. Fold in half to cover meat. Cut off excess dough to make a semi-circle and gently pinch the ends to seal. Carefully scoop with a spatula and place on a baking dish. Lightly brush the tops with oil. Bake for 20–30 minutes until dough appears light brown.

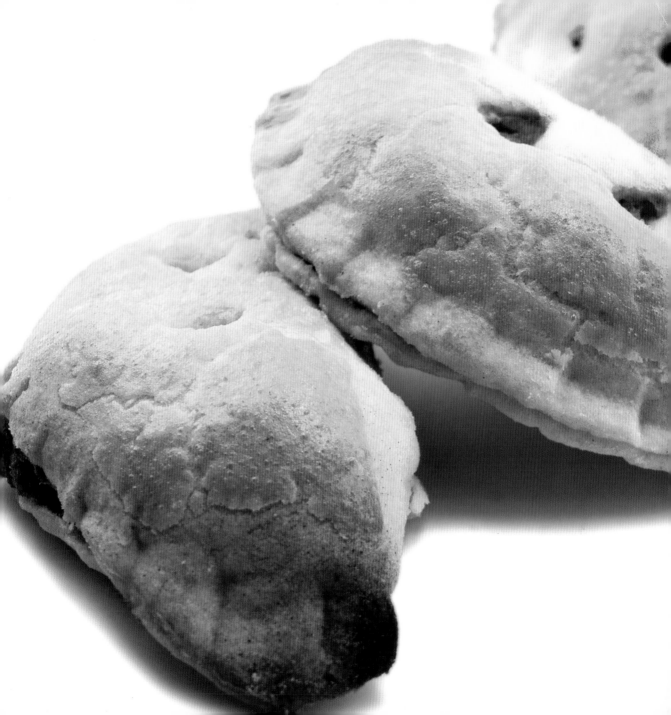

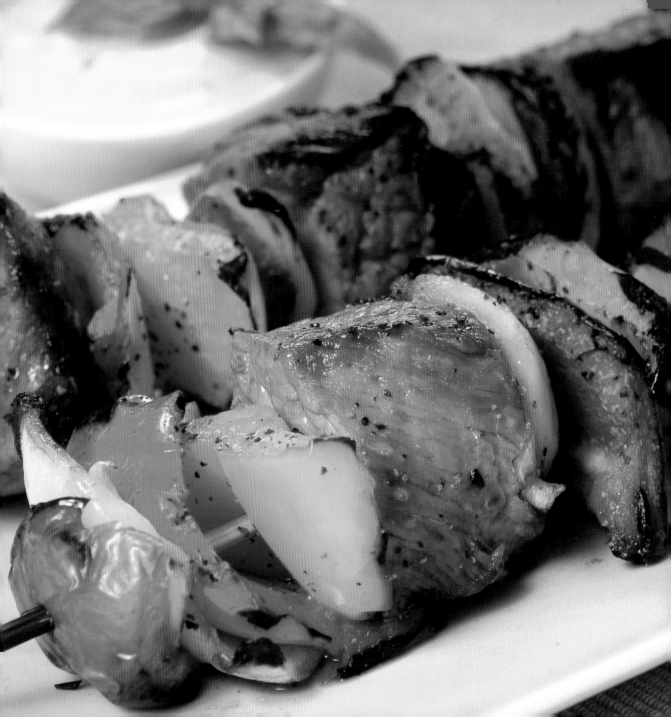

Kabobs with Raw Red Curry Sauce

KABOBS:

2   GRILLED BONELESS, SKINLESS
    CHICKEN BREASTS, CUBED
1   GREEN PEPPER, CUBED AND
    GRILLED

SAUCE:

1   CUP COCONUT MILK
1   SMALL RED BELL PEPPER, SLICED
3   GARLIC CLOVES
2   TABLESPOONS COLD-PRESSED
    OLIVE OIL
2   TABLESPOONS CURRY POWDER
1   TEASPOON SEA SALT

1. Alternate grilled chicken and green pepper on kabob sticks. Place the kabobs on serving plates and set aside. Combine sauce ingredients in a blender and blend on high speed until smooth. Scoop sauce with a ladle and pour over kabobs and onto the bottom of the plates.

Veggie Burgers

1 CUP COOKED PINTO BEANS,
  DRAINED AND RINSED
½ TEASPOON SALT
1 TEASPOON GROUND CUMIN
¼ CUP CILANTRO, CHOPPED
1 ONION, CHOPPED
1 GARLIC CLOVE, MINCED
1 CUP EACH OF CHOPPED BROCCOLI
  AND SPINACH
1 TABLESPOON CORNMEAL
1 TEASPOON OLIVE OIL

1. In a large bowl, coarsely mash the beans with a potato masher. Combine all other ingredients and stir until a thick dough forms. Use your hands to form burger patties. Cook for 5 minutes on each side on the grill or on a frying pan with light oil. Burgers should be firm and crusty.

Use a fork to eat and serve with a side of Sweet Potato Fries on page 113.

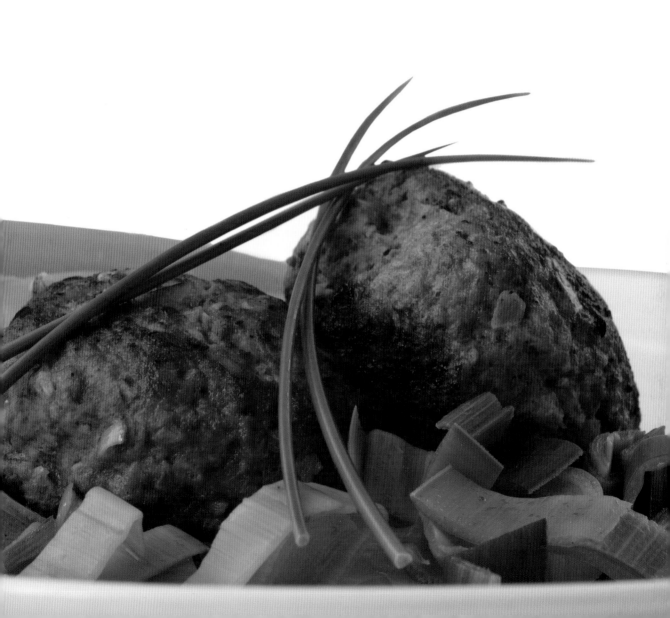

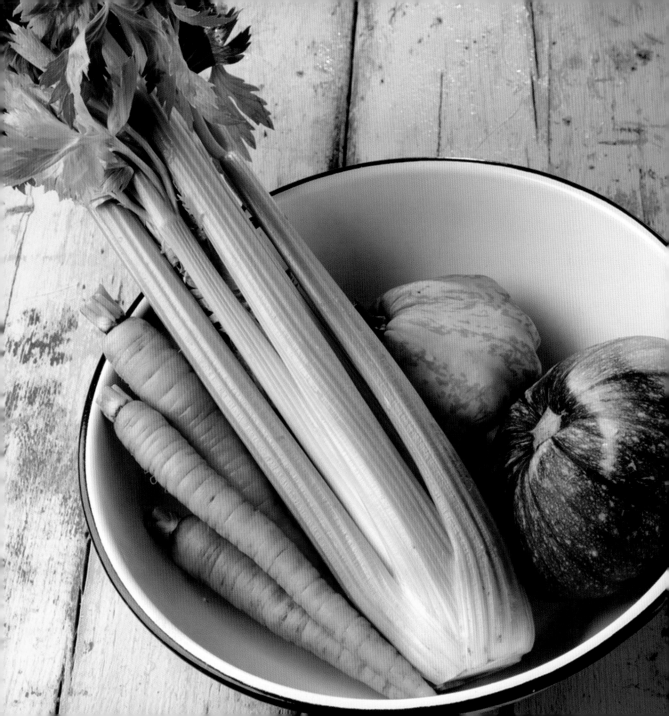

Soups, Sides, and Salads

Artichoke Bean Dip with Raw Spinach

1   14–16 OUNCE CAN OF WHITE BEANS,
    DRAINED AND RINSED
¼   CUP EXTRA VIRGIN OLIVE OIL
6   LARGE GARLIC CLOVES, SLICED
UP TO 2 CUPS CHICKEN BROTH OR
    WATER
3   OZ BABY SPINACH LEAVES
    (APPROXIMATELY TWO HANDFULS)
ONE 3–OZ JAR OF MARINATED
    ARTICHOKE HEARTS, DRAINED
SALT TO TASTE

1. Combine beans, olive oil, sliced garlic, and 1 cup of broth (or water) in a blender.

2. Blend until beans are smooth and creamy. Add broth or water ¼ cup at a time if the mixture is too dry.

3. Add spinach and artichoke hearts. Pulse several times until the spinach and artichoke are coarsely chopped and mixed into the dip.

Use this as a dip for tortilla chips.

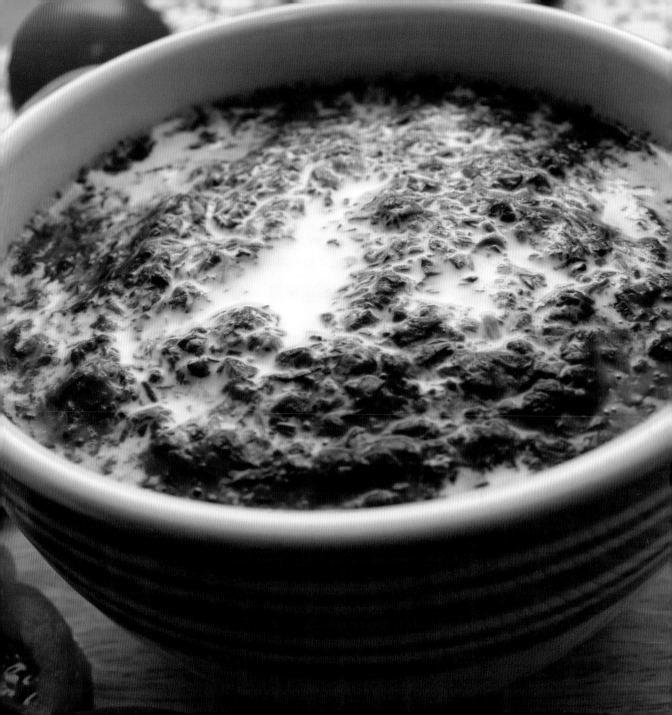

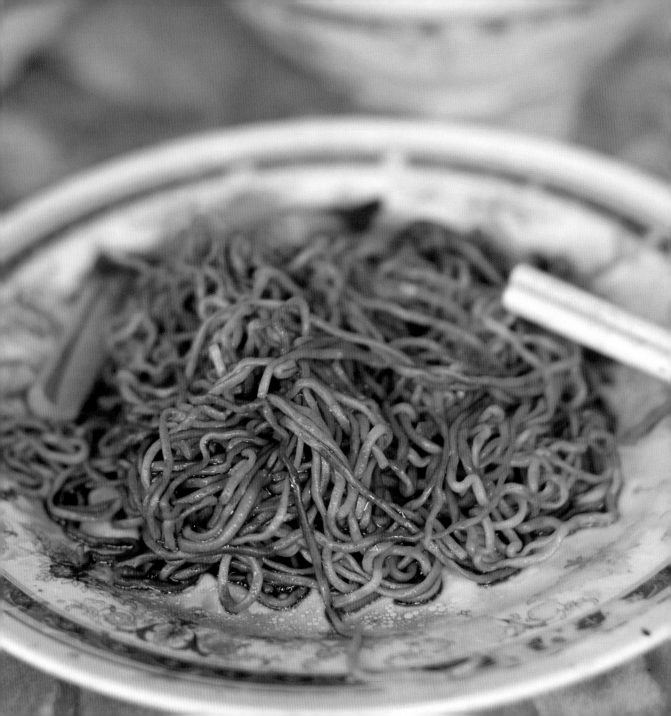

Asian Noodles

1   LB CORN SPAGHETTI
½   CUP LIGHT SESAME OIL
SWEETENER—1 TABLESPOON
     EVAPORATED CANE JUICE OR AGAVE
     NECTAR
1   TEASPOON SALT
1   TEASPOON BALSAMIC VINEGAR OR
     APPLE CIDER VINEGAR
1   GARLIC CLOVE, MINCED
1   SCALLION, SLICED
½   CUP ROASTED SESAME SEEDS

1. Boil spaghetti until tender. Do not over cook.

2. Rinse in cold water. Drain all excess water. Place spaghetti in a large bowl and set aside.

3. Combine all other ingredients and stir with a whisk until blended. Pour over spaghetti and toss.

Authentic Mango Salsa (Raw)

4   LARGE, RIPE TOMATOES, CUBED
1   LARGE, RIPE MANGO, PEELED AND
    CUBED
4   GARLIC CLOVES, MINCED
1   MEDIUM RED ONION, CHOPPED
2   WHOLE SCALLIONS, CHOPPED
2   CUPS FRESH CILANTRO LEAVES,
    CHOPPED
½   TEASPOON SEA SALT
1   TEASPOON GROUND CUMIN
1   TEASPOON GROUND CORIANDER
    JUICE OF 1 LARGE LEMON

1. Combine all ingredients, except lemon juice, in a large bowl.

2. Stir gently until ingredients are well distributed.

3. Squeeze lemon over the top.

4. Chill and serve with tortilla chips.

For a smoother texture, pulse 4–5 times in a food processor.

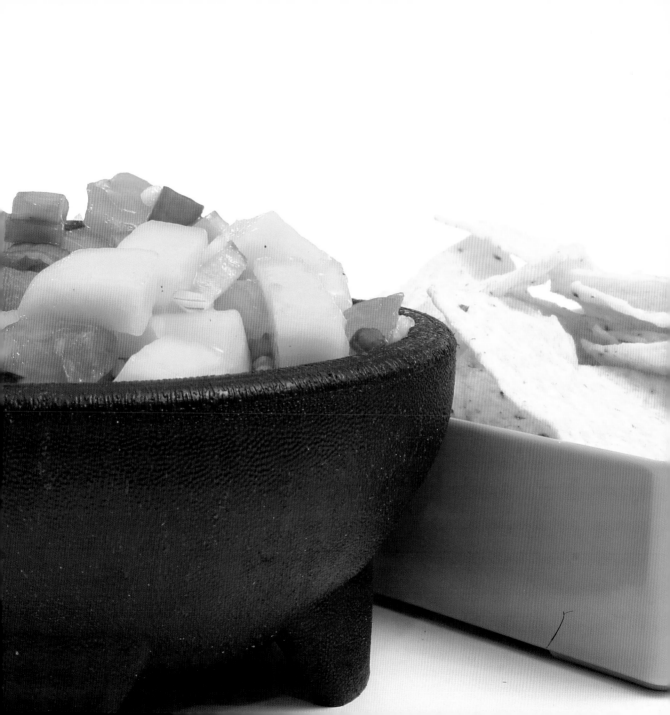

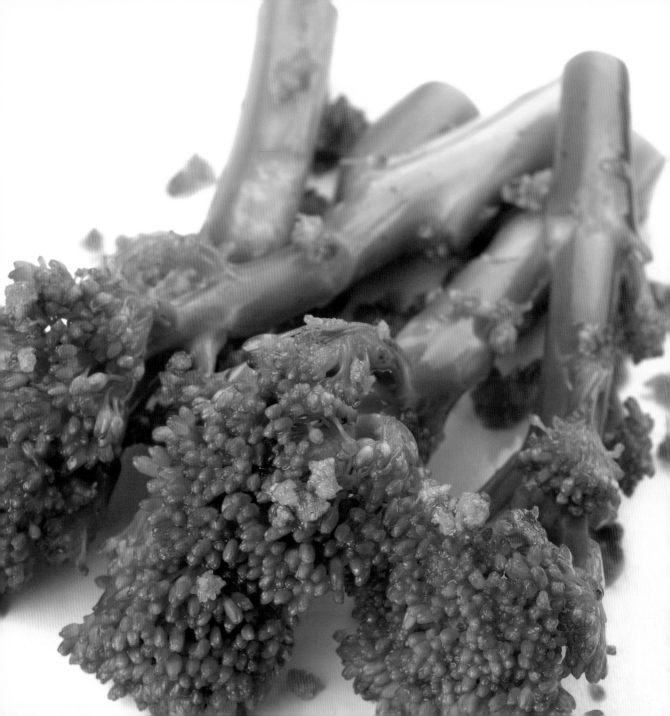

Broccoli Salad (Raw)

1 LB BROCCOLI CROWNS
½ CUP CORN OR CANOLA OIL
4 TABLESPOONS APPLE CIDER
    VINEGAR
1 TEASPOON SALT
SWEETENER—3 TABLESPOONS
    EVAPORATED CANE JUICE OR RAW
    AGAVE NECTAR
1 TABLESPOON FRESH GINGER,
    PEELED AND FINELY CHOPPED,
    OR 1 TEASPOON GROUND GINGER
    POWDER
1 CUP DRIED CRANBERRIES
¼ CUP RAW SESAME SEEDS OR RAW
    PUMPKIN SEEDS

1. Wash broccoli crowns thoroughly. Drain and set aside.

2. Combine oil, vinegar, salt, sweetener, and ginger in a large bowl. Blend thoroughly with a large whisk until sugar is dissolved.

3. Pour broccoli into bowl with oil and vinegar. Stir with a large spoon.

4. Add cranberries and seeds. Stir until blended.

5. Chill and serve.

Add cooked, chopped bacon if desired.

Chicken Salad

2 LARGE BONELESS, SKINLESS
   CHICKEN BREASTS   .
½ CUP CORN OR CANOLA OIL
¼ CUP APPLE CIDER VINEGAR
½ CUP GREEN PEPPER, FINELY
   CHOPPED
½ CUP CELERY, FINELY CHOPPED
3 TABLESPOONS ONIONS, FINELY
   CHOPPED
1 TABLESPOON SWEET RELISH
SALT AND PEPPER TO TASTE

1. Lightly season chicken with salt and pepper and cook thoroughly.

2. Finely shred chicken in a blender by pulsing several times.

3. Place chicken in a bowl and add oil, vinegar, green pepper, celery, onion, and relish.

4. Stir with a fork until blended.

5. Add salt and pepper to taste and chill.

Place chicken salad over a bed of lettuce and serve with corn chips.

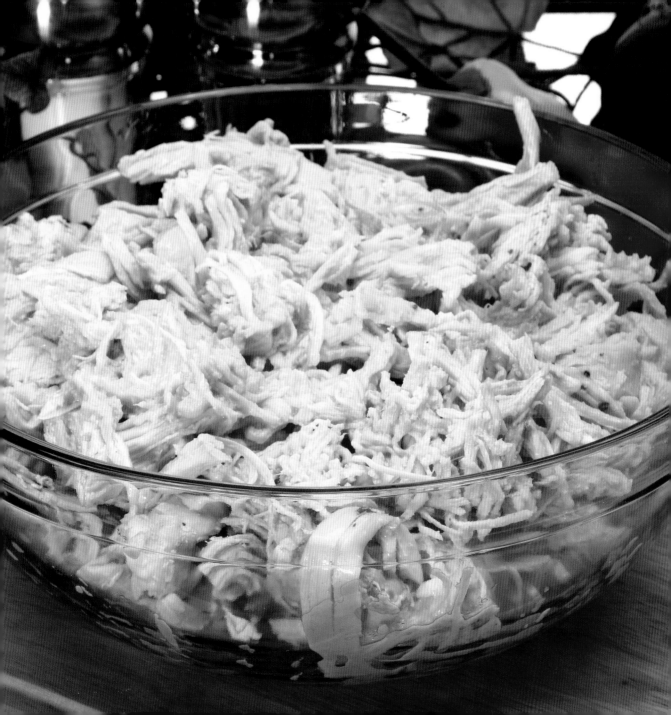

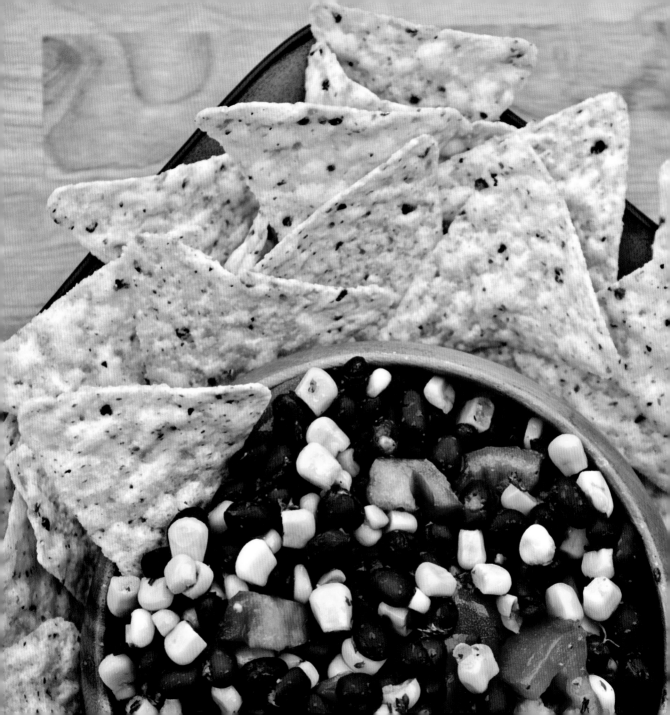

Cool Beans

2 CUPS BLACK BEANS, COOKED AND
RINSED
1 CUP CILANTRO, CHOPPED
1 SCALLION, FINELY CHOPPED
1 SMALL ROMA TOMATO, CHOPPED
½ CUP CORN KERNELS
½ TEASPOON GROUND CUMIN
JUICE OF 1 SMALL LIME

1. Combine all ingredients in a medium bowl. Toss gently. Chill and serve with tortilla chips.

Cool Cucumber Soup (Raw)

2 CUPS CUCUMBER, CHOPPED
1 CUP ZUCCHINI, CHOPPED
1 CUP AVOCADO, PEELED AND
   CHOPPED
JUICE OF 1 LARGE LEMON
1 SMALL GARLIC CLOVE, MINCED
2 TABLESPOONS COLD-PRESSED
   OLIVE OIL
½ TEASPOON SALT
3 CUPS LUKEWARM WATER

1. Blend all ingredients in a blender until smooth.

2. Serve cold or at room temperature.

Top with a thin slice of lime and a mint leaf.

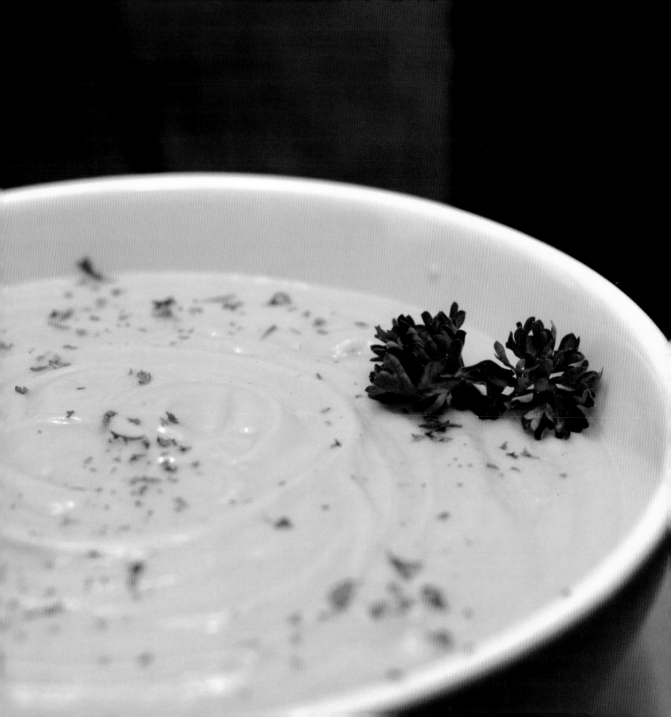

Corn Bread Stuffing

6 STALE CORN BREAD MUFFINS
  (FROM RECIPE ON PAGE 129)
¼ CUP CELERY, CHOPPED
¼ CUP GREEN PEPPER, CHOPPED
¼ CUP ONION, CHOPPED
1 GARLIC CLOVE, CHOPPED
2 TABLESPOONS EXTRA VIRGIN OLIVE
  OIL
CHICKEN OR TURKEY BROTH
SALT AND BLACK PEPPER TO TASTE

1. Bake cornbread muffins until medium brown. Cool completely and leave uncovered at room temperature until stale. If time permits, cover loosely and refrigerate overnight.

2. Preheat oven to 400°F.

3. Use your hands to crumble the corn bread into a large baking dish. Set aside.

4. Combine celery, green pepper, onion, garlic, and olive oil in a small saucepan. Simmer and stir until brown.

5. Pour vegetables into corn bread mixture.

6. Add broth while stirring, until corn bread is submerged.

7. Add salt and pepper to taste.

8. Bake on the middle rack of the oven until top and sides become crusty and stuffing becomes firm (approximately 45 minutes).

Serve with Chicken or Beef Gravy on page 220.

Corn Relish

3 CUPS CORN KERNELS
1 CUP CHOPPED ONION
1 CUP CHOPPED CUCUMBER
2 CUPS TOMATO, DICED
2 CUPS RAW APPLE CIDER VINEGAR
1 TABLESPOON SALT
2 TEASPOONS TURMERIC
2 CUPS AGAVE NECTAR OR
  EVAPORATED CANE JUICE
2 CUPS WATER

1. Combine all ingredients in a medium-sized pot. Bring to a boil, cover, and simmer until vegetables are soft (approximately 25 minutes). Cool completely. Place in a covered container and chill for several hours. Use a slotted spoon to scoop. Serve cold over grilled chicken or toss into a salad.

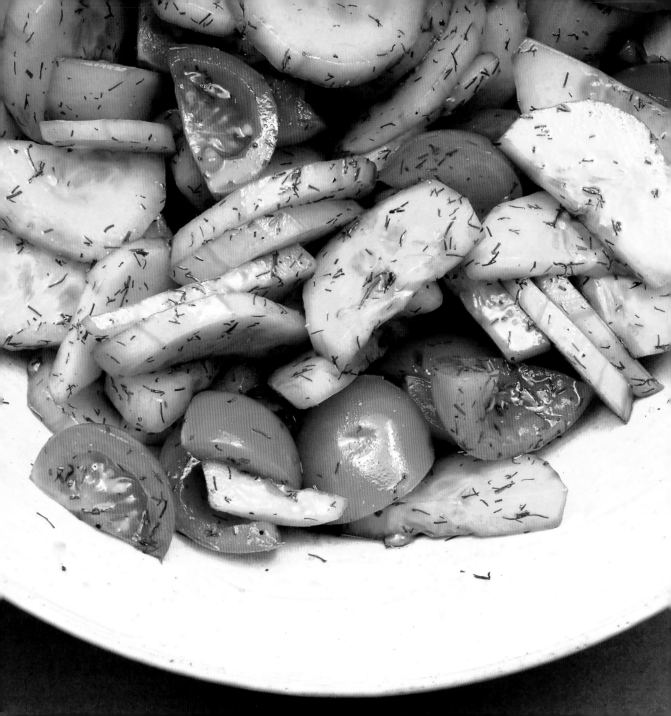

Cucumber Tomato Salad (Raw)

5   CHERRY TOMATOES, CUT INTO
    QUARTERS
1   LARGE CUCUMBER, PEELED AND
    SLICED
1   CUP FRESH DILL, CHOPPED
JUICE OF 1 LARGE LEMON
1   TABLESPOON AGAVE NECTAR
¼   TEASPOON SALT

1. Combine all ingredients in a large bowl. Stir gently until blended. Cover and refrigerate until ready to serve. Stir before serving.

Fluffy Mashed Potatoes

3   LARGE RUSSET POTATOES
½   CUP EXTRA VIRGIN OLIVE OIL
1   GARLIC CLOVE, CHOPPED
2   TEASPOONS DRIED, CRUSHED
     THYME LEAVES
1   TEASPOON SALT
½   TEASPOON BLACK PEPPER
UP TO 1 CUP WARM WATER, CHICKEN
     BROTH, OR VEGETABLE BROTH

1. Peel and wash potatoes and cut into thirds.

2. Boil potatoes until soft. Drain excess water. Place in a large mixing bowl and set aside.

3. Combine olive oil, garlic, thyme, salt, and pepper in a small saucepan. Simmer over low heat. Stir constantly until brown.

4. Add garlic mixture to potatoes. Mash with a large fork until lumpy.

5. Add ½ cup of warm water or broth. Mix with an electric mixer at low speed.

6. Increase the mixer speed to medium. Mix and add liquid until potatoes are light and fluffy.

Top with Fried Onion Topping on page 219.

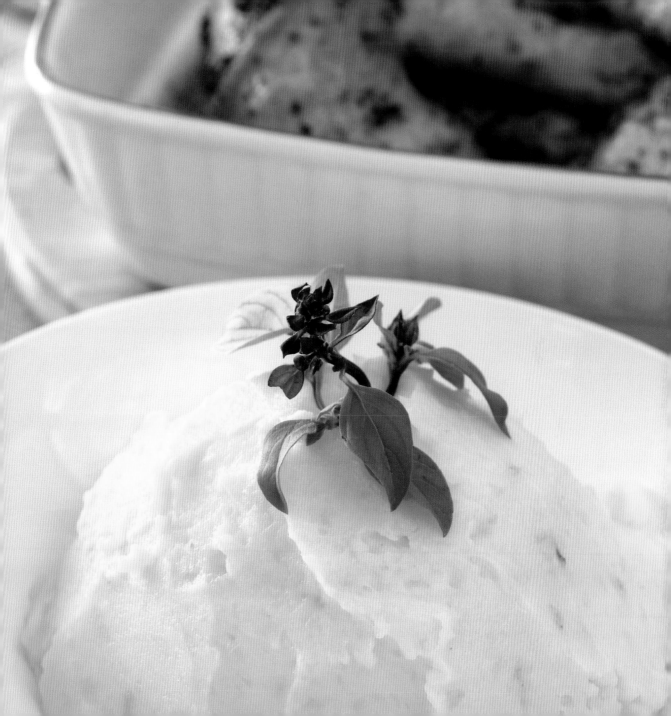

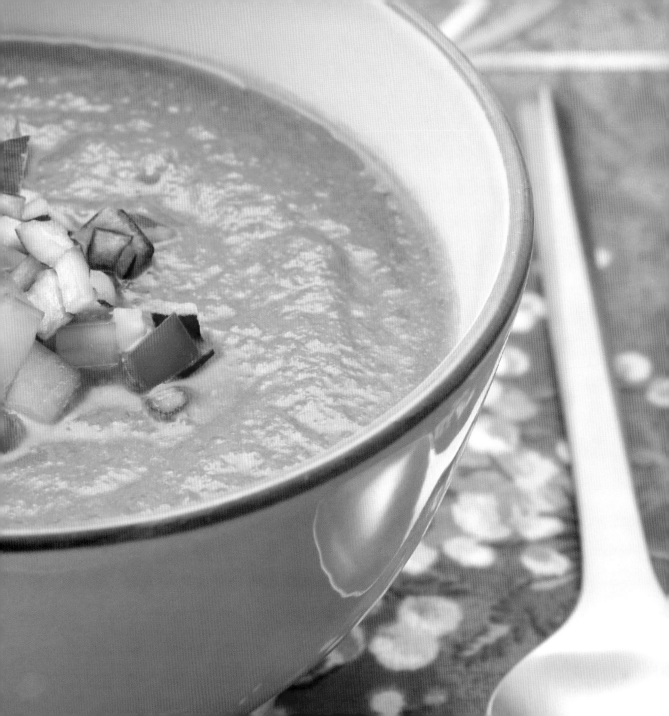

Gazpacho (Raw)

1   CUP WATER
½   CUP COLD-PRESSED OLIVE OIL
4   LARGE TOMATOES
1   LARGE GARLIC CLOVE
5   FRESH BASIL LEAVES
2   CUPS FRESH CILANTRO LEAVES
½   TEASPOON SEA SALT

TOPPING
1   MEDIUM AVOCADO, CUBED
1   SMALL CARROT, SHREDDED
1   SCALLION, SLICED

1. Combine all soup ingredients in a blender and blend until smooth.

2. Pour into individual bowls and add toppings to each.

3. Serve at room temperature or chilled.

Gazpacho can be eaten as a soup or used as a dip for vegetables or corn tortillas.

Hummus (Raw)

½ CUP SESAME OR PUMPKIN BUTTER
  FROM PAGE 221
1 SMALL ZUCCHINI
4 LARGE BLACK OLIVES
4 LARGE GREEN OLIVES
1 SMALL GARLIC CLOVE
2 TEASPOONS GROUND CUMIN
3 TABLESPOONS COLD-PRESSED
  OLIVE OIL
2 TEASPOONS SEA SALT
JUICE OF 1 SMALL LEMON

1. Combine all ingredients in a blender.

2. Blend at high speed until thick and creamy.

Serve as a dip with fresh carrot sticks or tortilla chips.

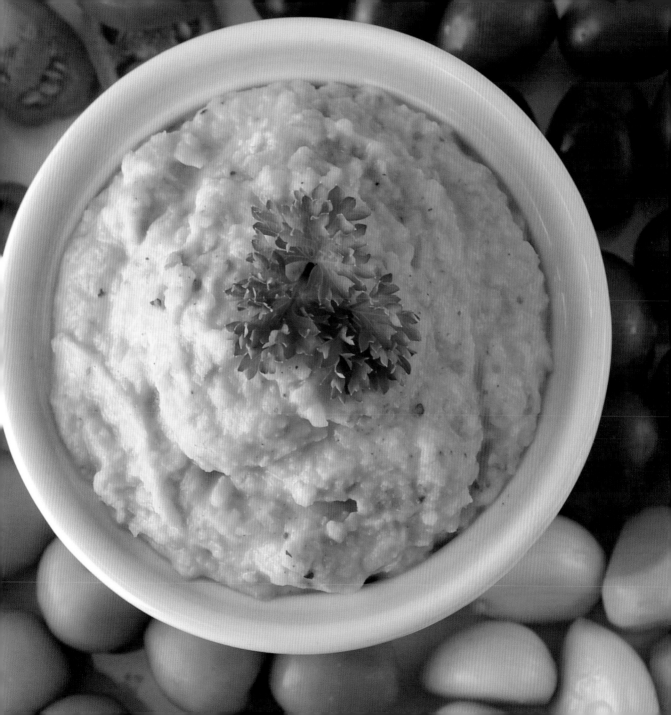

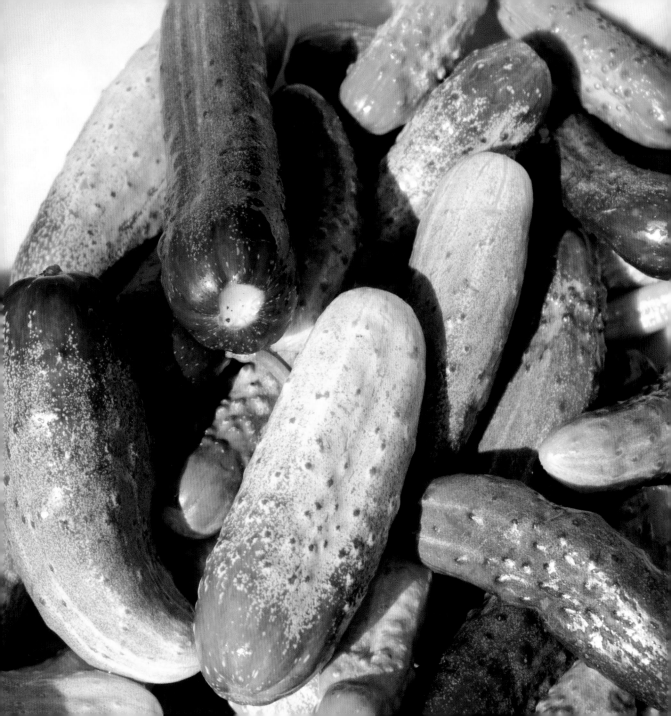

Korean Cucumber Kimchee (Raw)

10 KIRBY CUCUMBERS (ALSO CALLED PICKLING CUCUMBERS)
1 CUP SEA SALT
6 SMALL GARLIC CLOVES, MINCED
4 WHOLE SCALLIONS, SLICED
2 TABLESPOONS FRESH GINGER, PEELED AND FINELY CHOPPED
¼ CUP SESAME OIL
¼ CUP RAW SESAME SEEDS
CRUSHED RED PEPPER TO TASTE
1 TEASPOON RAW AGAVE NECTAR

1. Wash and slice cucumbers. Place in a large bowl.

2. Pour salt over cucumbers. Toss with your hands until the salt is evenly distributed.

3. Cover with a cloth. Set aside at room temperature for at least 2 hours. Salt will draw moisture out of the cucumbers.

4. Use a strainer to rinse the cucumbers under cold, running water. Keep rinsing until all the salt is removed. Taste frequently to test.

5. Use your hands to squeeze water from the cucumbers. Remove as much water as possible. Cucumbers will be limp.

6. Place cucumbers in a medium bowl and loosen with your hands. Add garlic, scallions, and ginger. Toss with a fork.

7. Use your fingertips to crush sesame seeds into a bowl.

8. Add agave and crushed red pepper to taste.

9. Chill and serve.

Serve with spiral corn pasta tossed in sesame oil.

The Autism Cookbook

Korean Dumpling Soup

BASE

8 CUPS OF CHICKEN OR BEEF BROTH
1 TABLESPOON ROASTED SESAME OIL
4 LARGE SCALLIONS FINELY CHOPPED
1 TABLESPOON DICED GINGER
SALT AND GROUND BLACK PEPPER TO
   TASTE
CRUSHED RED PEPPER TO TASTE
¼ CUP ROASTED, CRUSHED SESAME
   SEEDS

DUMPLING

½ CUP BUCKWHEAT FLOUR
½ CUP POTATO FLOUR
1 TEASPOON BAKING POWDER
½ CUP WATER
½ CUP CORN OR CANOLA OIL

1. Combine soup base ingredients in a large pot. Bring to a boil, lower the temperature, cover, and let simmer on low for 20 minutes.

2. Meanwhile, combine flours, water, and oil in a small bowl. Mix until well blended. The batter should be slightly thicker than pancake batter.

3. Scoop ¼ cup of batter at a time and pour into soup. Individual dumplings will form. Once all the batter is used, cover tightly and continue to simmer for five minutes.

Korean Seasoned Spinach (Raw)

1 LB BABY SPINACH LEAVES, THOROUGHLY WASHED
5 GARLIC CLOVES, MINCED
3 WHOLE SCALLIONS, SLICED
1 TABLESPOON FRESH GINGER, PEELED AND FINELY CHOPPED
SWEETENER—1 TEASPOON AGAVE NECTAR
½ TEASPOON SEA SALT
3 TABLESPOONS SESAME OIL
3 TABLESPOONS SESAME SEEDS
CRUSHED RED PEPPER TO TASTE

1. Bring 5 cups of water to a full boil in a large pot.

2. Dip spinach into water for 30 seconds. Remove promptly and place in a strainer.

3. Run spinach under cold water to cool completely.

4. Remove from running water; use your hands to squeeze water from the spinach. Remove as much water as possible. Spinach will be limp.

5. Place spinach in a small mixing bowl. Use your hands to toss and loosen the leaves.

6. Add garlic, scallions, ginger, sugar, salt, and sesame oil. Mix well with a fork.

7. Use your fingertips to crush sesame seeds into the bowl.

8. If desired, add crushed red pepper to suit your taste.

Serve with steamed quinoa or corn spaghetti tossed in sesame oil.

Mexican-Style Dip (Raw)

2 LARGE AVOCADOES, PEELED
2 TEASPOONS SALT
1 LARGE TOMATO, DICED
2 SCALLIONS, CHOPPED
1 SMALL RED ONION, CHOPPED
½ CUP FRESH CILANTRO LEAVES,
    CHOPPED
JUICE OF 1 SMALL LIME

1. Place avocadoes and salt in a medium bowl. Mash with a fork until smooth.

2. Mix in tomatoes, scallions, onions, and cilantro over the avocado.

3. Squeeze fresh lime juice over top.

Chill and serve with organic corn tortilla chips.

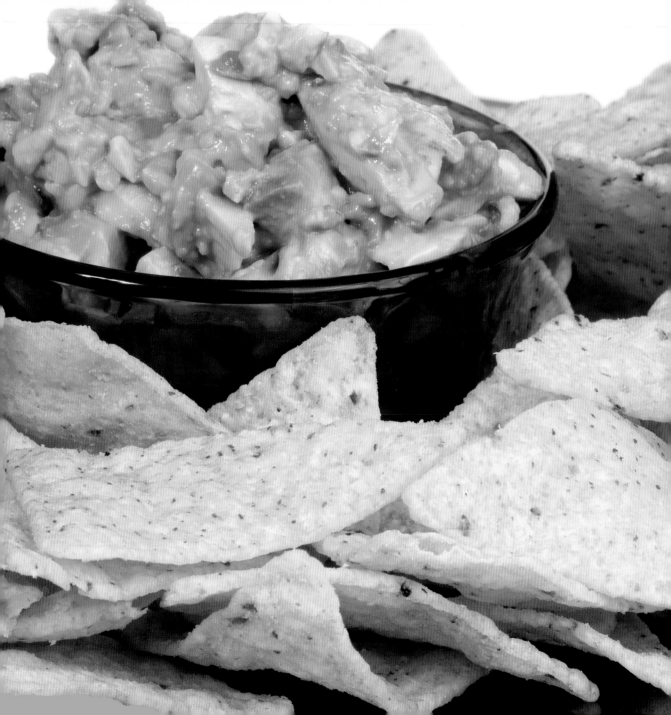

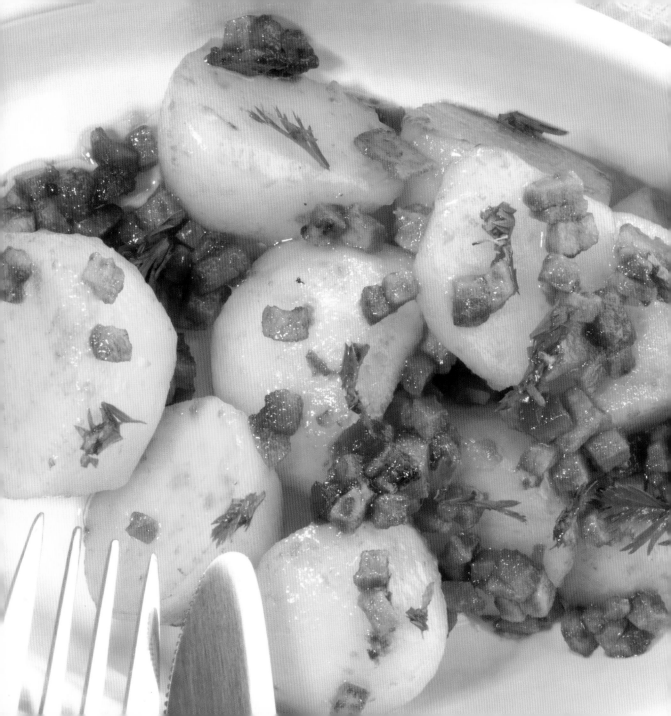

Potato Salad

3   LARGE RUSSET POTATOES
½   CUP CORN OR CANOLA OIL
¼   CUP APPLE CIDER VINEGAR
1   STRIP OF UNCURED PORK OR
    TURKEY BACON, COOKED AND
    CHOPPED
½   CUP GREEN PEPPER, FINELY
    CHOPPED
½   CUP CELERY, FINELY CHOPPED
1   TABLESPOON ONION, FINELY
    CHOPPED
SALT AND PEPPER TO TASTE
PAPRIKA AND SCALLIONS TO GARNISH

1. Peel potatoes. Wash and cut into bite-sized cubes.

2. Boil potatoes until slightly soft, not mushy. Drain and place in a large bowl. Cool completely.

3. Add oil, vinegar, bacon, green pepper, celery, and onion.

4. Stir gently with a large spoon until blended. Add salt and pepper to taste.

5. Garnish with paprika and chopped scallions.

6. Chill and serve.

Quinoa Chicken Salad

1   CUP QUINOA
2   CUPS WATER
¼   CUP CIDER-FLAX DRESSING (RECIPE
    ON PAGE 223)
1   SCALLION, CHOPPED
½   CUP STEAMED BROCCOLI
½   CUP DRIED CRANBERRIES
    (OPTIONAL)
1   CUP OF COOKED CHICKEN, CUBED
1   AVOCADO, PEELED AND SLICED

1. Bring water to a boil in a medium-sized pot. Add quinoa seeds. Reduce the temperature to a simmer, cover tightly, and cook for 15 minutes or until all water is dissolved. Cool completely.

2. Place in a large mixing bowl and add Cider Flax Dressing, scallions, broccoli, and cranberries. Toss vigorously until dressing is distributed.

3. Place in serving bowls. Top with chicken and avocado and serve.

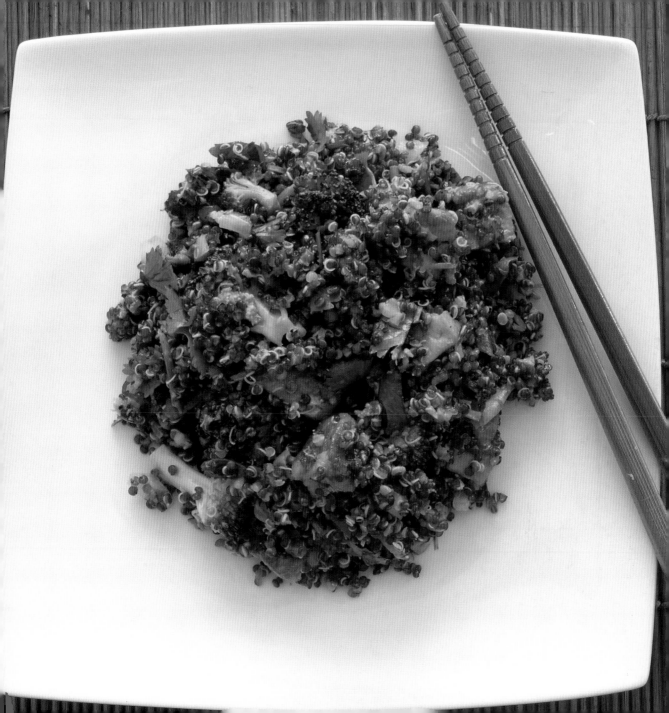

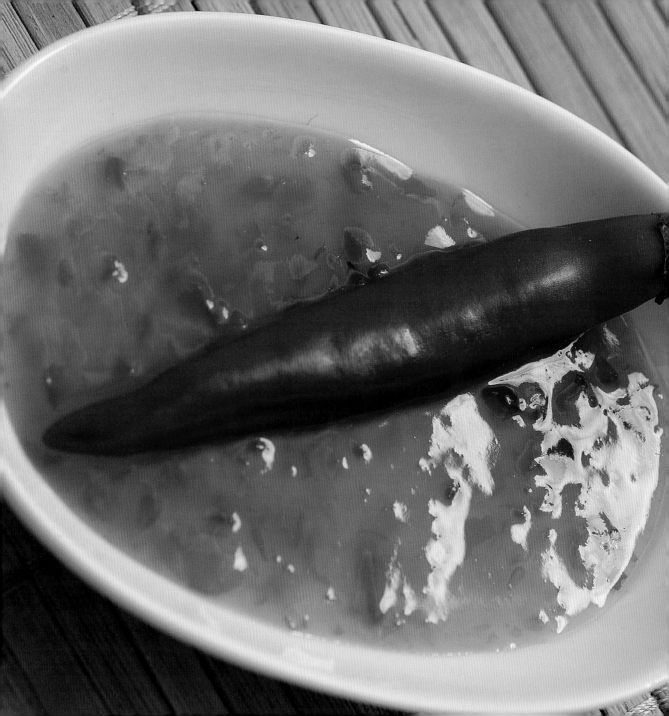

Quinoa Salad with Sweet Chili Sauce

1 CUP QUINOA SEEDS
2 CUPS WATER
1 RED BELL PEPPER, CHOPPED
2 SCALLIONS, MINCED
1 MEDIUM CARROT, SHREDDED
¼ CUP THAI SWEET CHILI SAUCE
SALT TO TASTE
½ CUP TOASTED PUMPKIN SEEDS,
   COARSELY CHOPPED
2 TABLESPOONS APPLE CIDER
   VINEGAR

1. Cook quinoa seeds in water on the stove top or in a rice cooker until all water is absorbed. Cool completely. Pour into a large bowl. Add the red bell peppper, scallions, carrot, and chili sauce and toss until blended. Mix in the pumpkin seeds. Toss in salt to taste. Serve chilled or at room temperature.

Rosemary Potatoes

5 MEDIUM-SIZED RED OR GOLDEN
   POTATOES
½ CUP EXTRA VIRGIN OLIVE OIL
3 GARLIC CLOVES, MINCED
½ TEASPOON DRIED, CRUSHED
   ROSEMARY LEAVES
2 TEASPOONS SALT
1 TEASPOON BLACK PEPPER

1. Preheat oven to 325°F.

2. Cover a cookie sheet with aluminum foil and set aside.

3. Wash potatoes thoroughly. Slice into wedges.

4. Combine potatoes, olive oil, garlic, rosemary, salt, and pepper in a large bowl.

5. Stir thoroughly with a large spoon.

6. Spread seasoned potatoes over the cookie sheet.

7. Place cookie sheet on the middle rack of the oven.

8. Bake for approximately 40 minutes or until potatoes are soft when pricked with a fork.

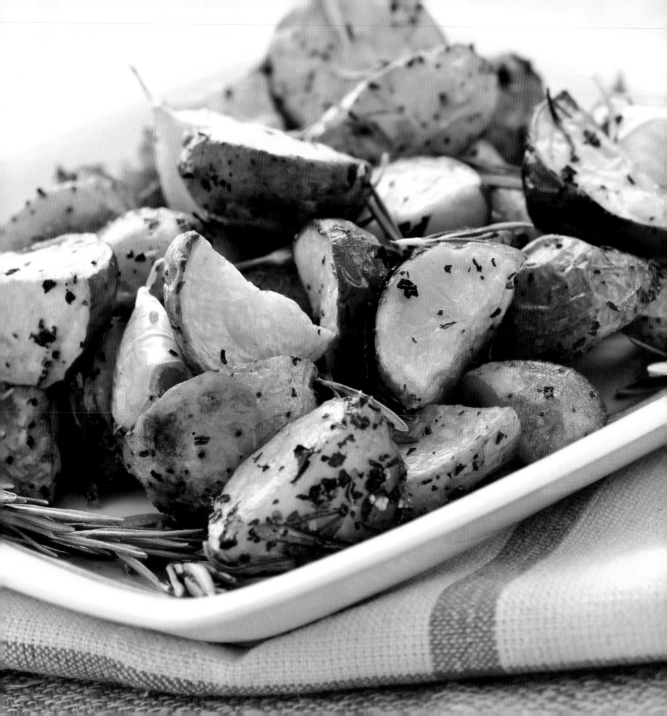

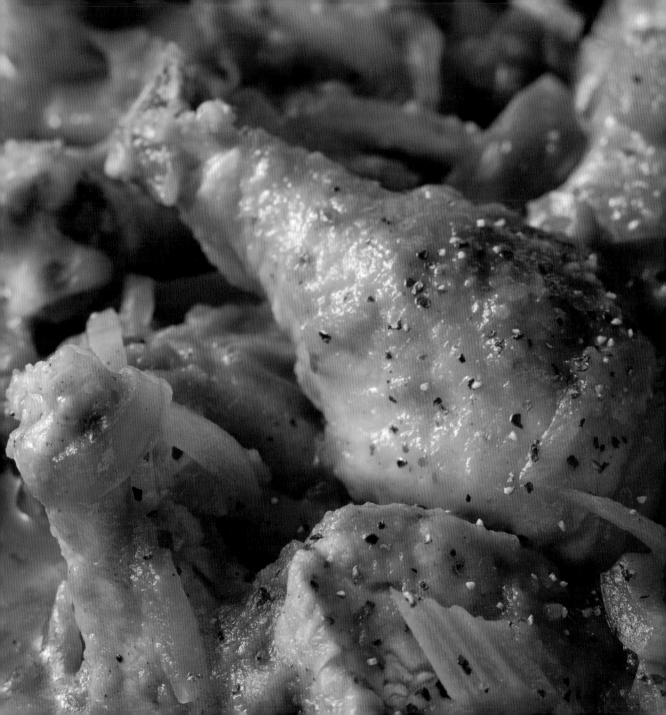

Sausage-Chicken Gumbo

¼ CUP OLIVE OIL
1 SMALL ONION, FINELY CHOPPED
4 GARLIC CLOVES, FINELY CHOPPED
2 TEASPOONS CRUSHED THYME
1 TEASPOON EACH OF SALT AND
GROUND BLACK PEPPER
4 CUPS CHICKEN OR BEEF BROTH
1 LARGE TOMATO, DICED
2 CUPS FROZEN, CUT OKRA
½ POUND CHICKEN
2 CUPS KIELBASA SAUSAGE OR
OTHER SMOKED SAUSAGE, CUBED

1. Pour olive oil into a medium Dutch oven. Sauté the onion, thyme, salt, pepper, and garlic until vegetables are soft. Stir in broth, tomato, and okra. Cover and let simmer for 20 minutes. Stir in meats. Cover and simmer for an additional 20 minutes. Serve warm over a bed of steamed quinoa.

Simple Korean Stew

1 TABLESPOON OLIVE OIL
½ LB BEEF STEW MEAT
8 CUPS BEEF BROTH OR WATER
1 LARGE POTATO, PEELED AND CUBED
2 LARGE SCALLIONS, SLICED
1 SMALL ONION, SLICED
2 TABLESPOONS EACH OF MINCED
   GARLIC CLOVES AND GINGER
1 SMALL ZUCCHINI, SLICED INTO
   CIRCLES
TO TASTE: CRUSHED RED PEPPER,
   SALT, GROUND BLACK PEPPER, AND
   ROASTED SESAME SEEDS

1. In a large pot, heat olive oil and cook the beef until brown on all sides. Add water, scallion, onion, garlic, and ginger. Bring to a boil. Reduce the temperature to low, cover, and let simmer for 20 minutes. Open the lid and add zucchini and seasonings to taste. Cover and simmer for 15 minutes. Pour into serving bowls. Use your fingertips to crush sesame seeds over the stew and serve.

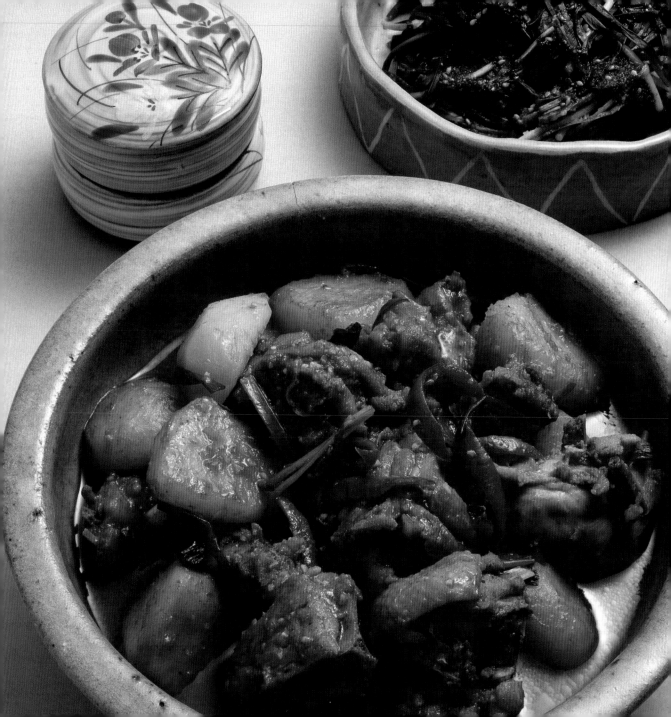

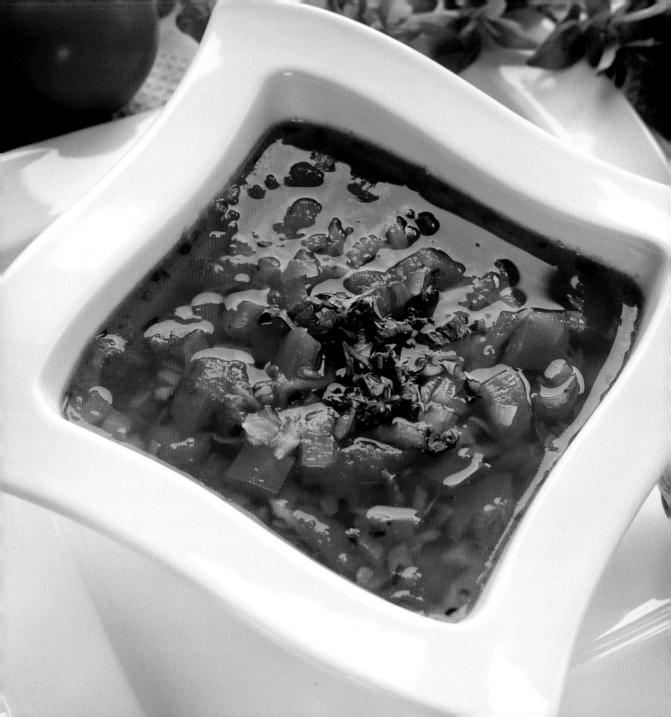

Slow Cooker Chicken Chili Soup

2 BONELESS, SKINLESS CHICKEN
   BREASTS CUT INTO CUBES
3 CUPS TOMATO, CUBED
½ CUP CORN KERNELS
3 CUPS CHICKEN BROTH
1 ONION, MINCED
2 GARLIC CLOVES, MINCED
1 TABLESPOON GROUND BLACK
   PEPPER
1 TABLESPOON CUMIN POWDER
SALT TO TASTE
1 CUP CILANTRO, CHOPPED

TOPPING
1 FRESH LIME
TORTILLA CHIPS
SLICED AVOCADO

1. Place all ingredients in a crock pot. Stir until well
   blended. Set temperature to medium heat, cover,
   and cook for 5–6 hours. Pour into bowls and top with
   tortilla chip pieces and lime juice.

Steamed Quinoa or Buckwheat with Veggies
(a yummy substitute for rice pilaf)

2 TABLESPOONS OLIVE OIL

½ CUP EACH OF CELERY, ONION, CARROT, AND GREEN PEPPER, CHOPPED

1 TEASPOON SALT

2 CUPS WATER OR BROTH

1 CUP WHOLE QUINOA SEEDS OR ROASTED BUCKWHEAT SEEDS

1. Heat olive oil over low heat in a medium pot.

2. Add all vegetables and salt. Stir frequently. Cook until brown.

3. Add water or broth to the pot. Increase heat, bringing the liquid to a boil.

4. Add quinoa or buckwheat seeds and stir until all ingredients are well blended.

5. Reduce heat to a low simmer. Cover tightly with a lid. Let simmer for 10 minutes or until water has soaked into the seeds.

6. Fluff with a fork prior to serving.

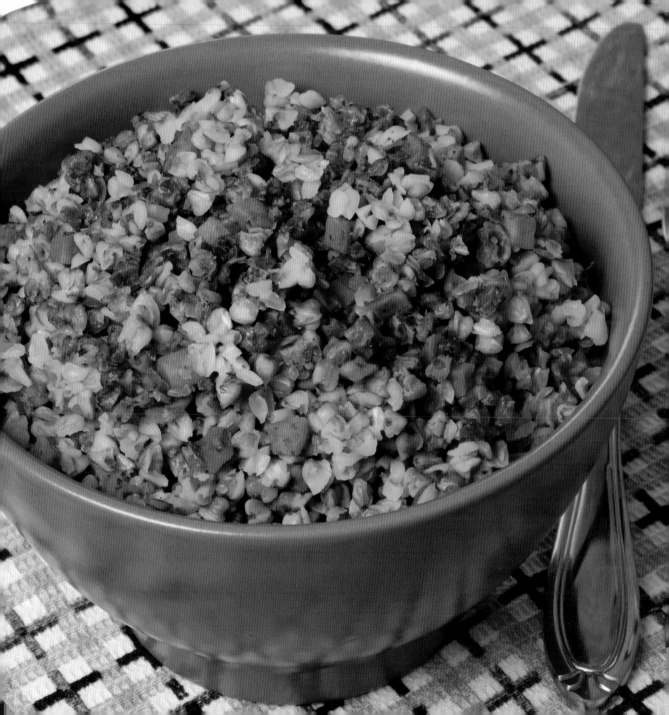

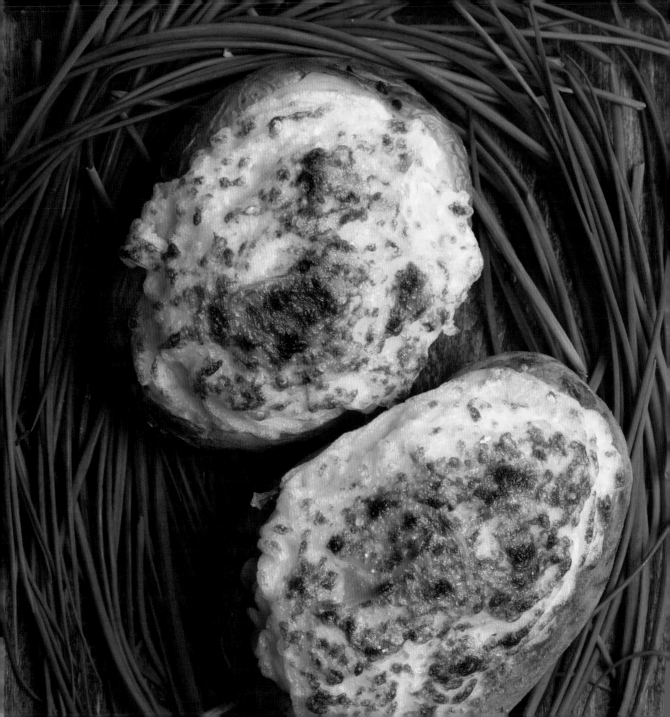

Stuffed Baked Potato

2   LARGE RUSSET POTATOES
¼   CUP OLIVE OIL
1   TEASPOON SALT
1   GARLIC CLOVE, MINCED
½   SMALL ONION, MINCED
ADDITIONAL OLIVE OIL

1. Preheat oven to 400°F.

2. Lightly oil potatoes. Place directly on the oven rack and bake for 1 hour. Turn halfway through cooking. Let cool completely.

3. Meanwhile, combine ¼ cup olive oil and onions and garlic in a small saucepan. Cook onions over low setting until very soft. Turn off heat and set aside.

4. Once cooled, slice potatoes in half, lengthwise. Scoop out potato filling, keeping shells intact. Place the filling in a small bowl.

5. Add the cooked onion mixture to the potato filling. Mix with an electric mixer on low speed until the mixture is smooth. Add olive oil by the teaspoon to loosen, if needed.

6. Spoon the potato mix back into the shells.

7. Bake at 400°F until tops of potatoes are crusty and light brown.

Sprinkle with bacon bits or chopped scallions. Serve warm.

The Autism Cookbook

Sweet Potato Casserole

2 LARGE SWEET POTATOES (OR YAMS)
½ CUP CORN OR CANOLA OIL
2 TEASPOONS GROUND CINNAMON
½ TEASPOON GROUND NUTMEG
2 TABLESPOONS LIGHT BROWN
   SUGAR
1 TEASPOON SALT (OPTIONAL)
UP TO 1 CUP WARM WATER
2 CUPS MINIATURE MARSHMALLOWS

1. Bake potatoes until soft, or peel, slice, and boil potatoes until soft.

2. Preheat the oven to 400°F.

3. Place potatoes in a large mixing bowl. Add oil, cinnamon, nutmeg, brown sugar, and salt to the potatoes. Mash with a large fork until lumpy.

4. Add ½ cup of warm water. Mix with an electric mixer at low speed.

5. Increase the mixer speed to medium. Add water by the tablespoon until potatoes are light and fluffy.

6. Pour potatoes into a baking dish and spread marshmallows evenly over top.

7. Bake for approximately 10 minutes or until marshmallows appear slightly brown.

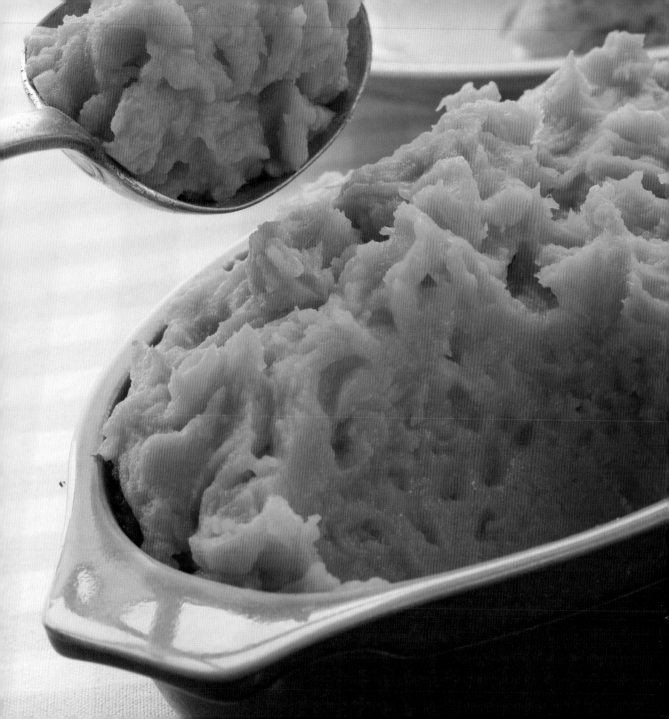

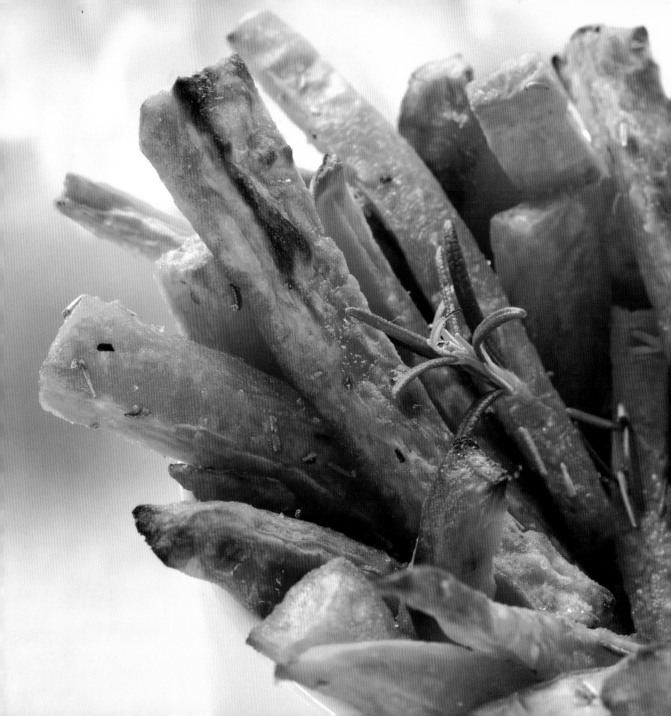

Sweet Potato Fries

1 LARGE SWEET POTATO, PEELED IF
  DESIRED
1 TABLESPOON OLIVE OIL
1 TEASPOON EACH OF NUTMEG,
  GARLIC POWDER, AND SALT
PINCH OF GROUND CLOVE (OPTIONAL)

1. Wash and pat dry the sweet potato. Cut into slices and place in a medium mixing bowl. Add oil and seasonings. Stir until blended. Place the slices in a single layer, on a non-stick baking dish. Bake 30–40 minutes until potatoes are light brown on the edges.

Thai Coconut Soup (Raw)

MEAT AND "MILK" OF 1 LARGE COCONUT
1   SMALL GARLIC CLOVE
2   TABLESPOONS OLIVE OIL
1   TABLESPOON FRESH GINGER,
    FINELY CHOPPED
2   CHERRY TOMATOES
¼   CUP GREEN PEPPER, CHOPPED
JUICE OF 1 LARGE LEMON
¼   CUP EACH OF FRESH BASIL AND
    CILANTRO LEAVES, CHOPPED

1. Blend coconut meat and milk in a blender until smooth.

2. Add all remaining ingredients and blend again until smooth.

3. Serve at room temperature or warmed very slightly.

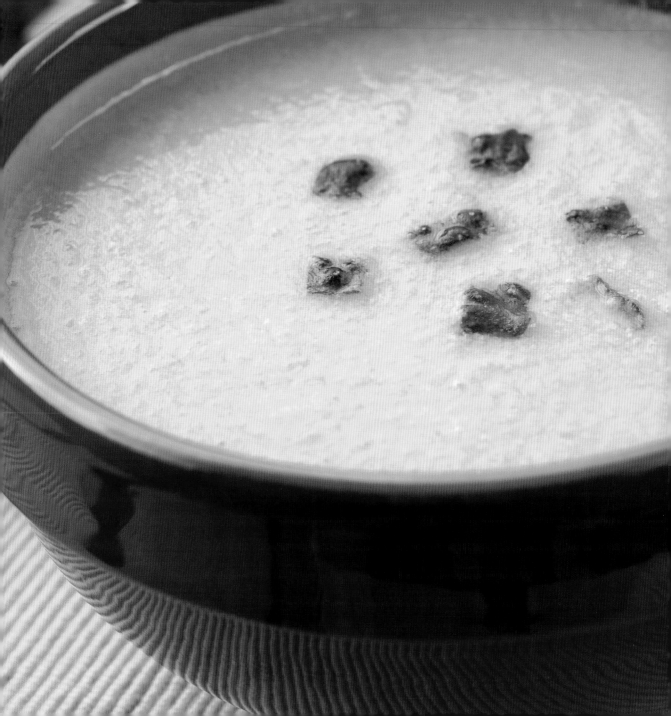

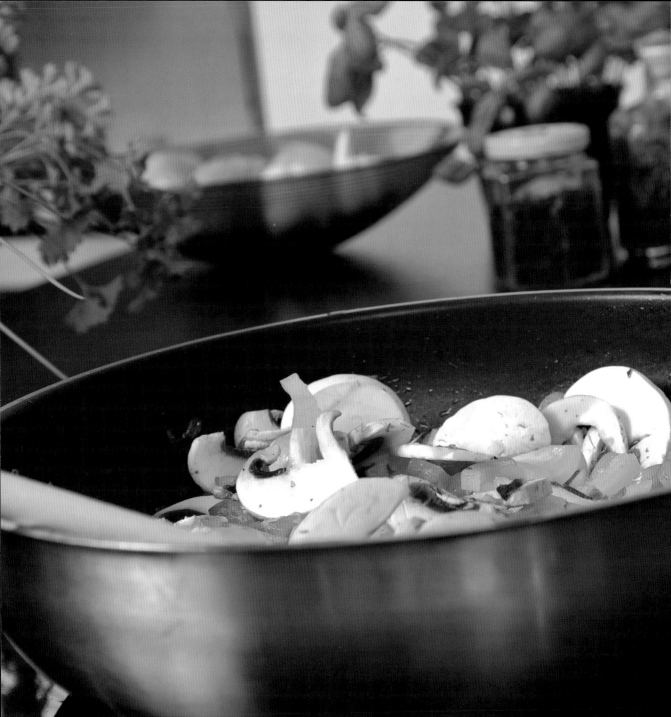

Vegetable Stir-Fry

5   LARGE MUSHROOMS, SLICED
1   LARGE ONION, SLICED
1   LARGE RED PEPPER, SLICED
½   LARGE ORANGE OR YELLOW
    PEPPER, SLICED
½   LARGE GREEN PEPPER, SLICED
½   LB FRESH BROCCOLI CROWNS
2   TABLESPOONS FRESH GINGER,
    PEELED AND FINELY CHOPPED
2   TABLESPOONS ROASTED SESAME
    SEEDS
¾   CUP EXTRA VIRGIN OLIVE OIL OR
    ROASTED SESAME OIL
1   TEASPOON SALT (OPTIONAL)

1. Combine all ingredients in a large mixing bowl. Stir until oil is distributed.

2. Preheat a large cast-iron skillet or wok to high temperature. Do not add extra oil.

3. Add vegetables to the skillet or wok. Toss frequently for 2 minutes. For softer vegetables, cook for 5 minutes.

4. Serve immediately.

Serve with grilled chicken.

The Autism Cookbook

Zesty Pasta Salad

3 CUPS SPIRAL CORN PASTA
1 PACKET DRY ITALIAN SALAD
   DRESSING MIX
½ CUP CORN OR CANOLA OIL
½ CUP RAW CIDER VINEGAR
1 MEDIUM CARROT, PEELED AND
   CHOPPED
1 SMALL GREEN PEPPER, CHOPPED
1 CUP BROCCOLI CROWNS, CHOPPED
SLICED GRILLED CHICKEN (OPTIONAL)

1. Boil pasta until cooked. Drain and rinse with cold water. Set aside.

2. Combine dressing mix, oil, and vinegar in a large mixing bowl. Whisk salad dressing until blended.

3. Add pasta, vegetables, and chicken. Toss until blended.

4. Chill and serve.

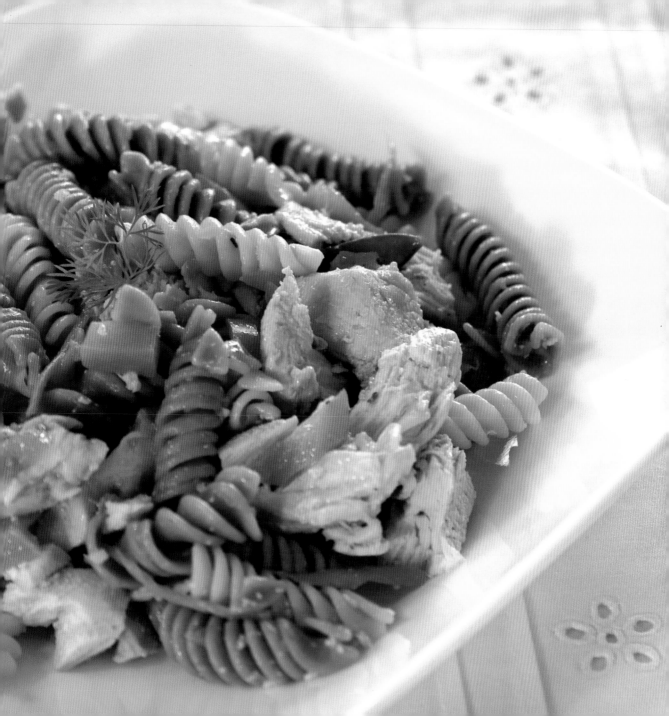

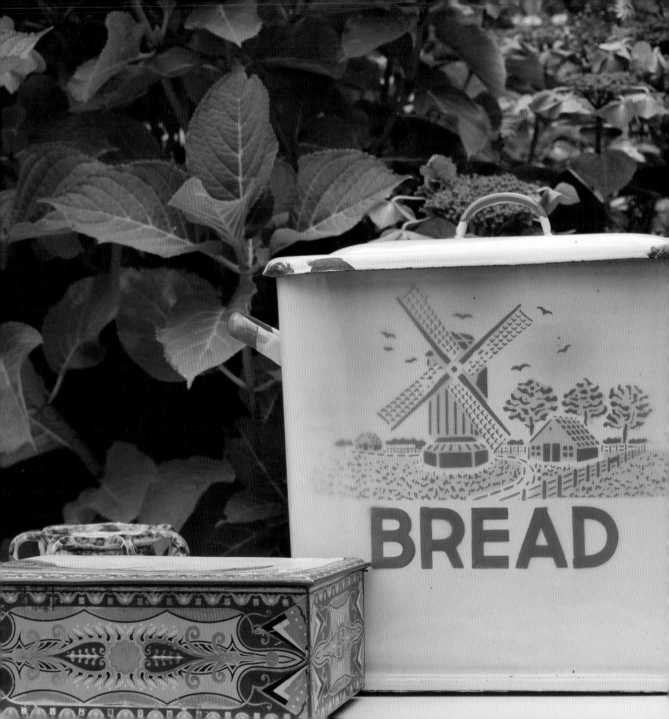

Whole-Grain Breads

The Autism Cookbook

Apple Bread

2   CUPS BUCKWHEAT FLOUR
1   TABLESPOON BAKING POWDER
    (ALUMINUM-FREE)
2   TABLESPOONS GROUND CINNAMON
¼   TEASPOON SALT
1   CUP UNSWEETENED APPLESAUCE
2   CUPS PEELED, CHOPPED APPLES
1½ CUPS LUKEWARM WATER
1   CUP CORN OR CANOLA OIL
SWEETENER—1½ CUPS RAW OR WHITE
    SUGAR OR 2 CUPS AGAVE NECTAR

1. Preheat oven to 400°F.

2. Combine flour, baking powder, cinnamon, and salt in a large mixing bowl. Sift thoroughly with a fork.

3. Add applesauce, chopped apples, water, oil, and sweetener. Mix with a large spoon until well blended.

4. Pour mixture into a non-stick, 9 x 5-inch loaf pan.

5. Bake on the middle rack of the oven until top appears light brown and slightly crusty (approximately 40–50 minutes).

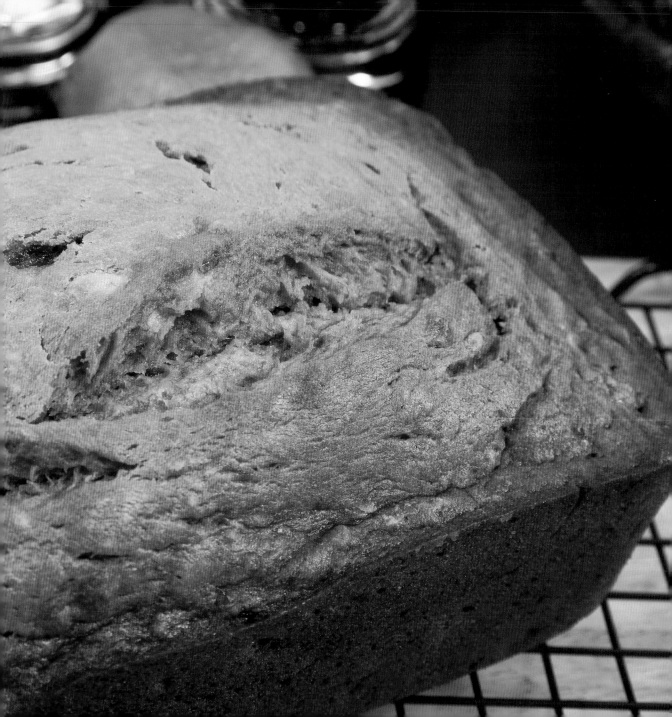

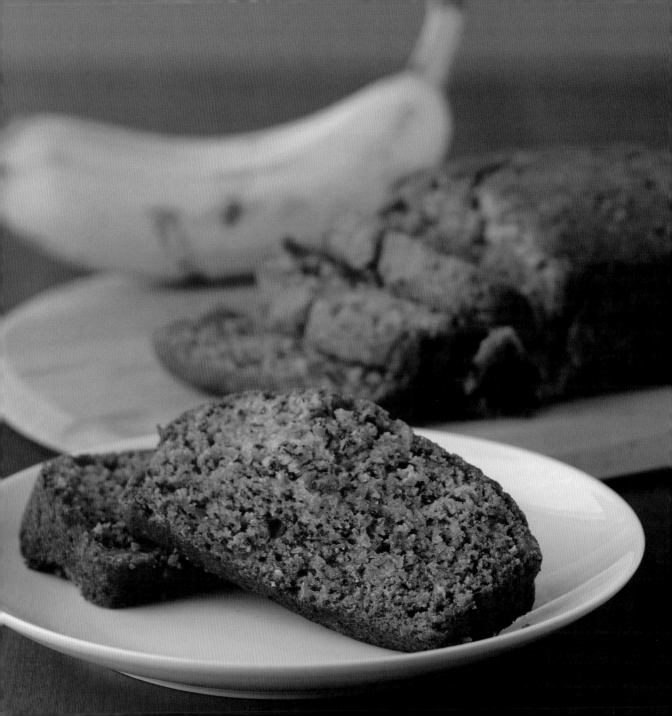

Banana Bread

2 CUPS BUCKWHEAT FLOUR

1 TABLESPOON BAKING POWDER
(ALUMINUM-FREE)

2 TABLESPOONS GROUND CINNAMON

¼ TEASPOON SALT

1 CUP UNSWEETENED APPLESAUCE

1 LARGE, VERY RIPE, MASHED
BANANA

½ CUP LUKEWARM WATER

¾ CUP CORN OR CANOLA OIL

1 TEASPOON GLUTEN-FREE VANILLA
EXTRACT

SWEETENER—1 ½ CUPS EVAPORATED
CANE JUICE OR AGAVE NECTAR

1. Preheat oven to 400°F.

2. Combine flour, baking powder, cinnamon, and salt in a large mixing bowl. Sift thoroughly with a fork.

3. Add applesauce, banana, water, oil, vanilla, and sweetener. Mix with a large spoon until well blended.

4. Pour mixture into a non-stick, 9 x 5-inch loaf pan.

5. Bake on the middle rack of the oven until top appears light brown and slightly crusty (approximately 40–50 minutes).

Cardamom Zucchini Bread

2   CUPS BUCKWHEAT FLOUR
1   TABLESPOON BAKING POWDER
1   TEASPOON SALT
¼   TEASPOON XANTHAN GUM
    (OPTIONAL)
2   TEASPOONS GROUND CARDAMOM
½   CUP AGAVE NECTAR OR
    EVAPORATED CANE JUICE
1   CUP WATER
¾   CUP CORN OR CANOLA OIL
1   CUP ZUCCHINI SQUASH, CHOPPED

1. Combine dry ingredients in a medium mixing bowl. Stir until blended. Add wet ingredients and zucchini. Mix well. Pour into a loaf pan and bake 45 minutes to 1 hour. Bread should be firm to the touch, crusty, and light brown.

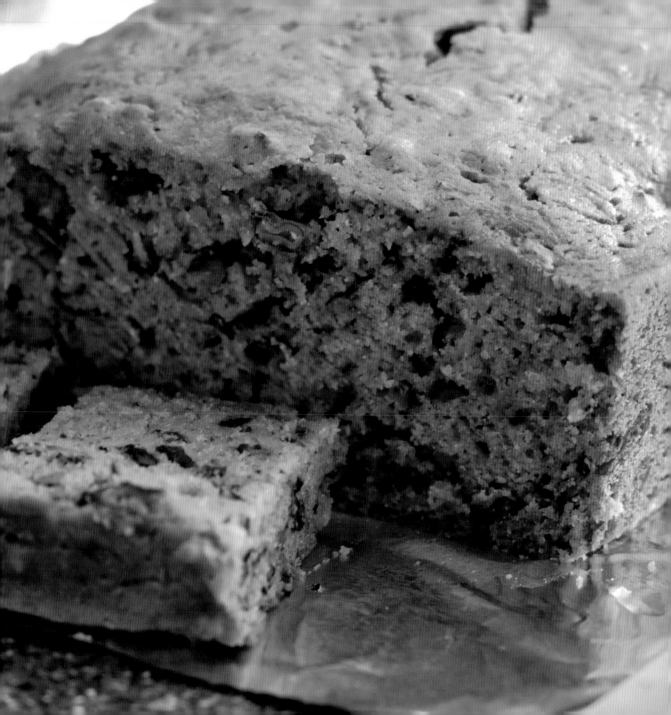

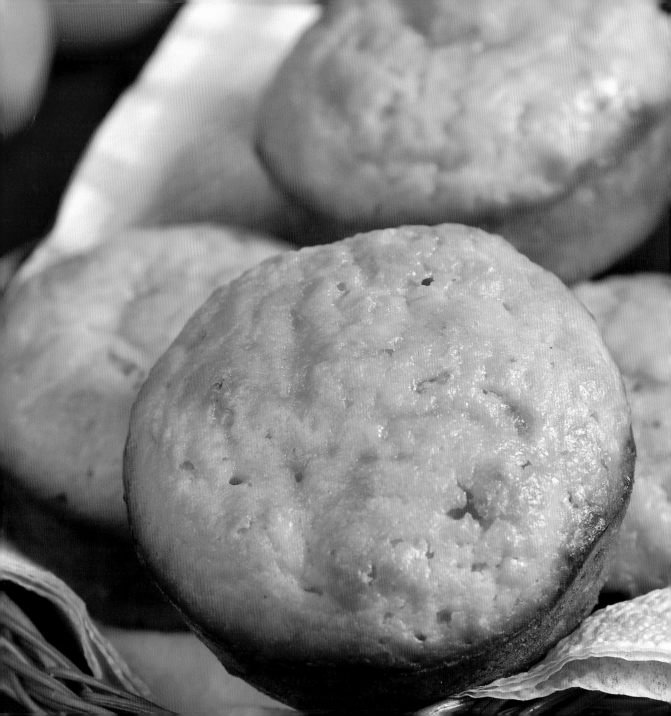

Corn Bread Muffins

2 CUPS CORN FLOUR OR CORNMEAL
¼ CUP BUCKWHEAT FLOUR
1 TEASPOON FLAX SEED MEAL (OPTIONAL)
2 TABLESPOONS BAKING POWDER (ALUMINUM-FREE)
¼ CUP UNSWEETENED APPLESAUCE
½ CUP CORN OR CANOLA OIL
2 CUPS WATER
1 TEASPOON SALT
SWEETENER—¼ CUP EVAPORATED CANE JUICE OR AGAVE NECTAR
WATER

1. Preheat oven to 400°F.

2. Combine flours, flax seed meal, and baking powder in a medium mixing bowl. Sift thoroughly with a fork.

3. Add applesauce, oil, water, and sweetener. Stir with a fork until a thick batter forms.

4. Spoon batter into muffin cups or use a 9-inch baking pan.

5. Bake on the middle rack of the oven for 10–15 minutes or until light brown.

Serve with Chunky Red Bean Chili on page 13. Also try with warm Sesame or Pumpkin "Butter" on page 221 or with fruit jam as a spread.

Ella's Italian Crackers (Raw)

1 CUP GOLDEN FLAX SEEDS
½ CUP EACH OF SWEET ONION AND
   RED BELL PEPPER
1 CUP CHOPPED TOMATOES
1½ TABLESPOONS FRESH LEMON JUICE
½ GARLIC CLOVE
1 STALK OF CELERY
1 TEASPOON EACH OF DRIED BASIL,
   OREGANO, AND SEA SALT

1. Use an Excalibur food dehydrator or preheat an oven to the lowest setting with the door ajar.

2. Place all ingredients in a food processor and process until uniform. Seeds will remain whole. Turn off the food processor, scrape down the sides, and process again. Entire processing time should be no more than one minute.

3. Use a spatula to spread the mixture evenly over a teflex sheet (non-stick dehydrator sheet) or use a 14 x 14-inch sheet of parchment paper for the oven.

4. Place the teflex sheet on a dehydrator tray or place the parchment paper on a baking tray.

5. Place in the dehydrator at 105°F or in the oven with the door ajar for five hours.

6. Remove the tray from the dehydrator or oven. Place the teflex or parchment sheet on the counter and score the crackers to your desired size.

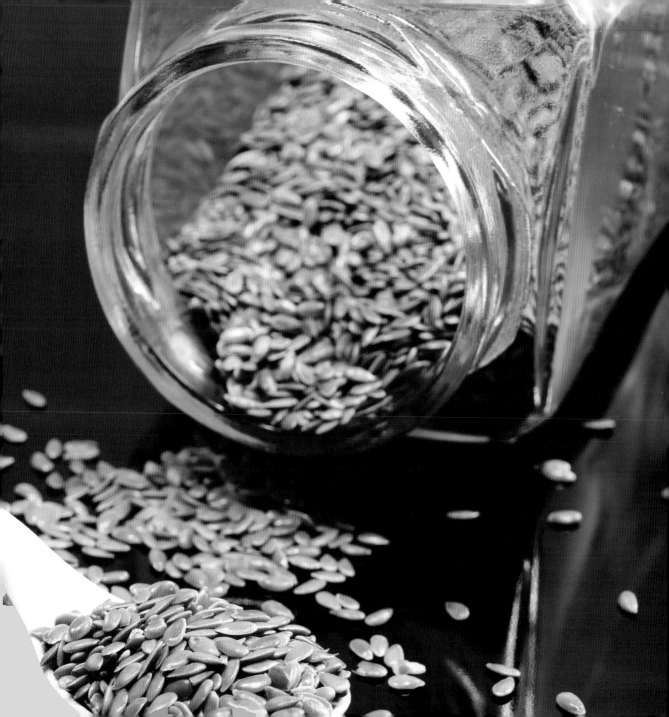

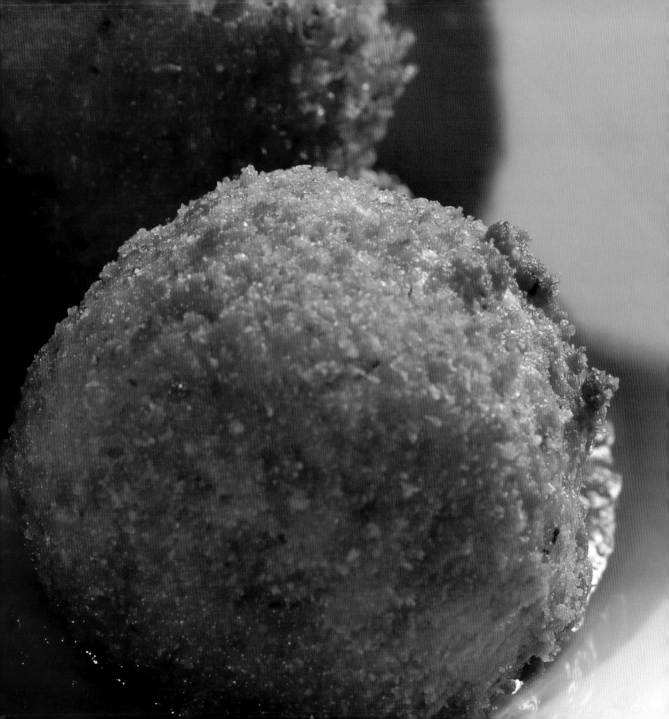

Hushpuppies

1 CUP CORN MEAL
½ TABLESPOON ALUMINUM-FREE
 BAKING POWDER
2 TEASPOONS SALT
1 TEASPOON EACH OF GARLIC
 POWDER AND GROUND BLACK
 PEPPER
¼ CUP CORN OR CANOLA OIL
¼ CUP WATER
1 FINELY CHOPPED ONION

1. Combine dry ingredients in a medium mixing bowl. Sift with a fork until blended. Add wet ingredients and the onion. Let the batter sit at room temperature for 15 minutes to thicken.

2. Heat corn or canola oil in a deep fryer. Use a large spoon to scoop 1 tablespoon of batter. Using the back of another spoon, scrape the batter into hot oil. Cook 5–7 hushpuppies at a time, until light brown.

Serve warm with Slow Cooker Barbecue Chicken on page 46.

Italian-Style Breadcrumbs

3 CUPS QUINOA FLAKES
1 TABLESPOON GARLIC POWDER
½ TEASPOON SALT
1 TABLESPOON DRIED, CRUSHED
   BASIL
1 TABLESPOON DRIED, CRUSHED
   OREGANO

1. Combine all ingredients in a bowl. Stir until all ingredients are well blended.

2. Heat a medium skillet to a low setting. Pour the mixture into the warm skillet. Toss constantly until very lightly browned.

3. Remove from heat and let cool completely.

Use in Meatloaf and Party Meatball recipes.

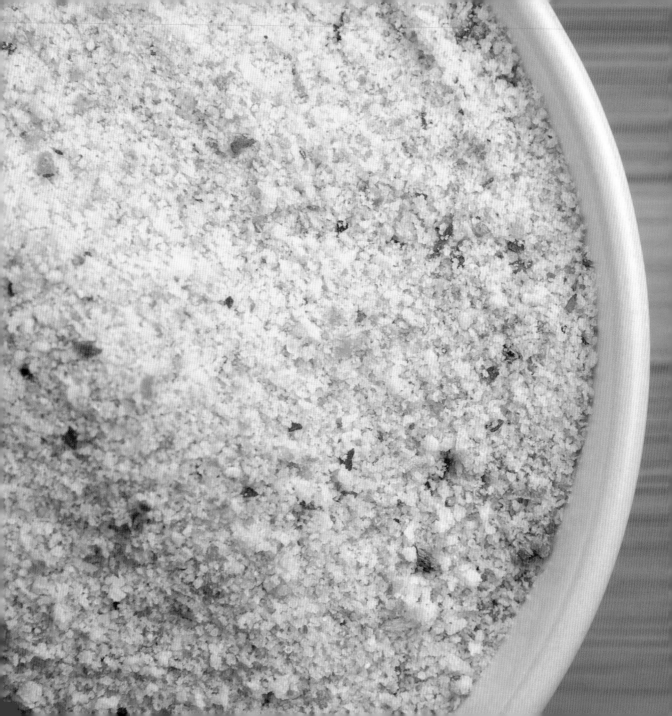

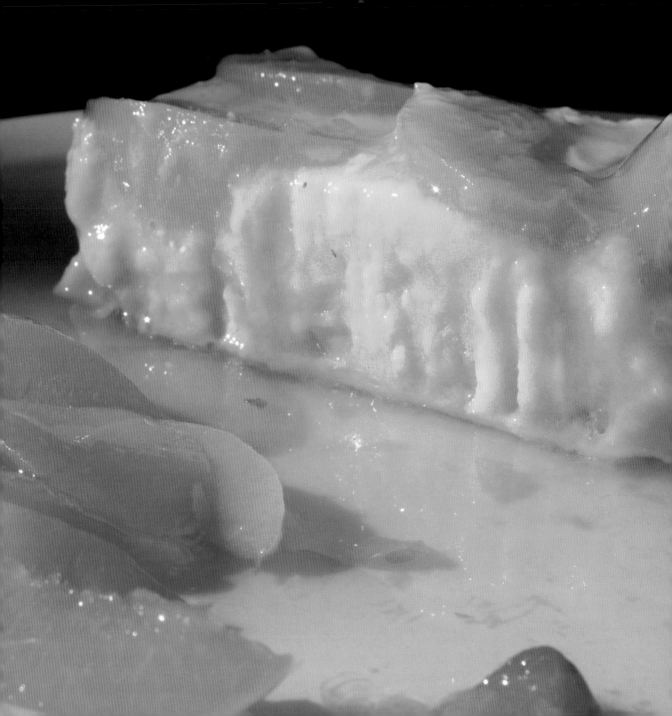

Peachy Corn Bread

1 CORNBREAD RECIPE FROM PAGE 129
1 LARGE PEACH, PEELED AND SLICED
  OR 1 CAN OF SLICED PEACHES,
  DRAINED

1. Preheat oven to 400°F. Lightly oil the bottom of a
   9-inch round baking dish. Prepare Corn Bread recipe
   and pour into the baking dish. Arrange the fruit on
   top of batter. Bake for 30 minutes or until sides of
   the cornbread are crusty. Cool completely, slice, and
   serve directly from the baking dish.

Pumpkin Bread

2 CUPS BUCKWHEAT FLOUR
1 TABLESPOON BAKING POWDER
   (ALUMINUM-FREE)
2 TABLESPOONS GROUND CINNAMON
1 TEASPOON EACH OF GROUND
   NUTMEG AND GROUND CLOVE
¼ TEASPOON SALT
1 CUP UNSWEETENED APPLESAUCE
1 CUP FULLY COOKED, MASHED
   PUMPKIN
½ CUP LUKEWARM WATER
¾ CUP CORN OR CANOLA OIL
SWEETENER—1 ½ CUPS EVAPORATED
   CANE JUICE OR AGAVE NECTAR

1. Preheat oven to 400°F.

2. Combine flour, baking powder, cinnamon, nutmeg, clove, and salt in a large mixing bowl. Sift thoroughly with a fork.

3. Add applesauce, pumpkin, water, oil, and sweetener. Mix with a large spoon until well blended.

4. Pour mixture into a non-stick, 9 x 5-inch loaf pan.

5. Bake on the middle rack of the oven until top appears light brown and slightly crusty (approximately 40–50 minutes).

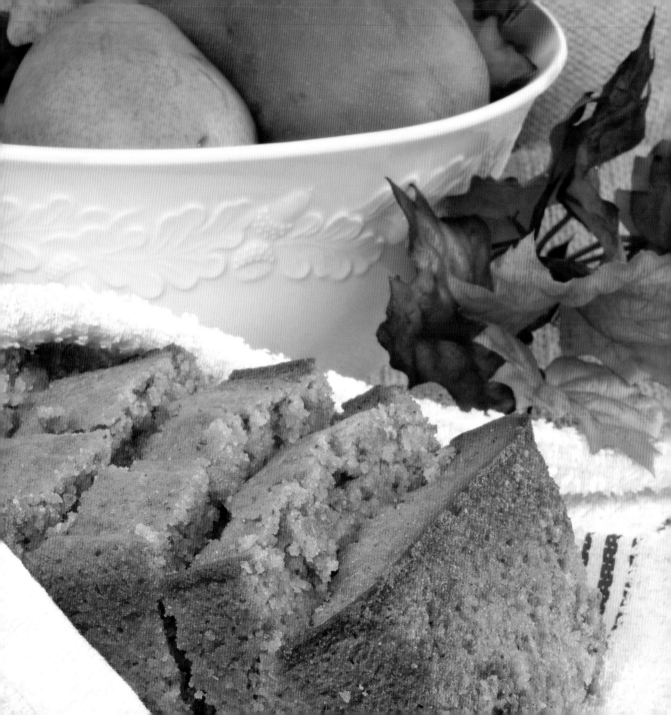

Veggie Corn Bread Muffins

2   CUPS CORN FLOUR OR CORNMEAL

¼   CUP BUCKWHEAT FLOUR

1   TEASPOON FLAX SEED MEAL
    (OPTIONAL)

2 TABLESPOONS BAKING POWDER
    (ALUMINUM-FREE)

½   CUP CORN OR CANOLA OIL

2   CUPS WATER

1   TEASPOON SALT

SWEETENER—¼ CUP EVAPORATED
    CANE JUICE OR AGAVE NECTAR

1   TABLESPOON EACH OF FINELY
    CHOPPED ZUCCHINI, GREEN
    BELL PEPPER, AND RED BELL
    PEPPER

2   TABLESPOONS CORN KERNELS

1. Preheat oven to 400°F.

2. Combine flours, flax seed meal, and baking powder in a medium mixing bowl. Sift thoroughly with a fork.

3. Add oil, water, and sweetener. Stir with a fork until a thick batter forms.

4. Add vegetables and mix well.

5. Spoon batter into muffin cups.

6. Bake on the middle rack of the oven for 10–15 minutes or until muffins become light brown.

Wholesome Fruit and Seed Bread

1   CUP LUKEWARM WATER
½   CUP CORN OR CANOLA OIL
SWEETENER—½ CUP EVAPORATED
    CANE JUICE OR AGAVE NECTAR
2   CUPS BUCKWHEAT FLOUR, PLUS
    ADDITIONAL FOR DUSTING
2   TEASPOONS SALT
¼   CUP EACH OF DRIED CRANBERRIES,
    RAW SUNFLOWER SEEDS, AND RAW
    PUMPKIN SEEDS

TOPPING
2   TABLESPOONS PURE HONEY OR
    AGAVE NECTAR

1. Preheat oven to 400°F.

2. In a large bowl, combine lukewarm water, oil, and sweetener. Stir until sweetener is well blended. Set aside.

3. In a medium bowl, combine flour, salt, cranberries, and seeds. Stir with a fork until well blended.

4. Slowly add flour mixture to water/oil mixture while stirring. Keep adding flour until a clean ball of dough forms. Dust with additional flour if dough is too loose.

5. Knead dough with your hands for 1 minute. Shape dough into an oval ball and place in a loaf pan.

6. Place loaf pan on the middle rack and bake for approximately 40 minutes or until light brown.

7. Let cool completely.

8. Brush a thin layer of honey or agave nectar over the bread.

If desired, lightly roast your seeds on the stove top using a light oil and salt. Allow seeds to cool prior to adding to the dough.

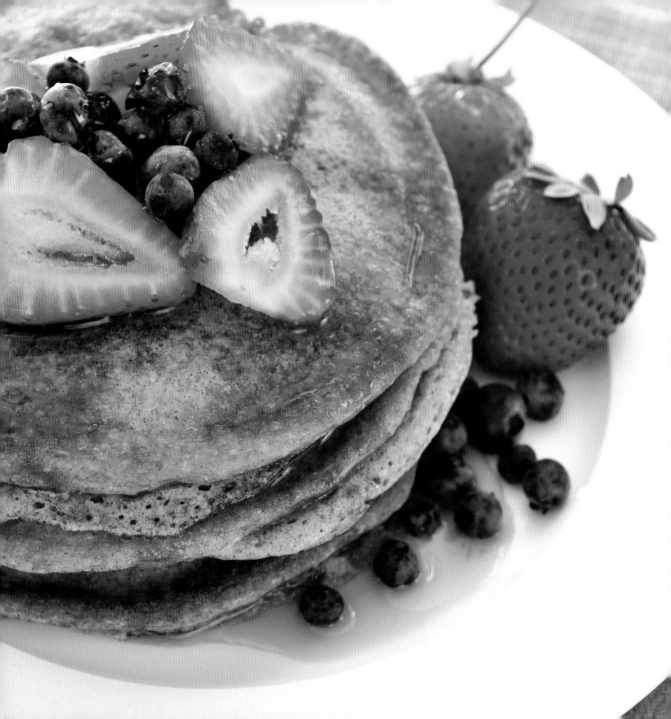

Breakfast Items

The Autism Cookbook

Apple Cinnamon Quinoa

2   CUPS WATER
½   CUP APPLE, PEELED AND CHOPPED
1   TEASPOON SALT
2   TABLESPOONS AGAVE NECTAR
¾   CUP QUINOA FLAKES
GROUND CINNAMON TO TASTE

1. In a medium pot, bring water to a boil. Stir in apples, salt, and agave nectar. Reduce heat to medium and let simmer for 2 minutes. Stir in quinoa flakes and cinnamon. Reduce heat to low and stir for 1 minute. Remove from heat and allow the cereal to thicken. Serve warm. If desired, top with raisins, sliced bananas, or pure maple syrup.

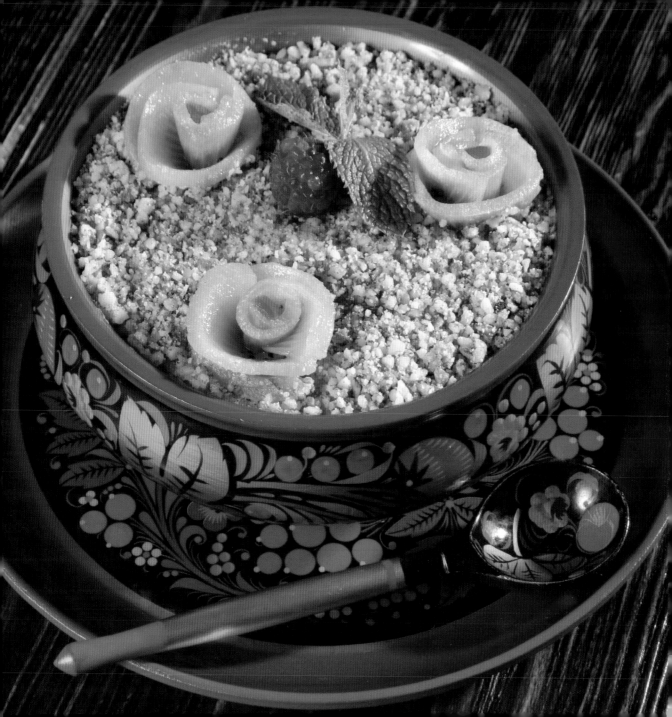

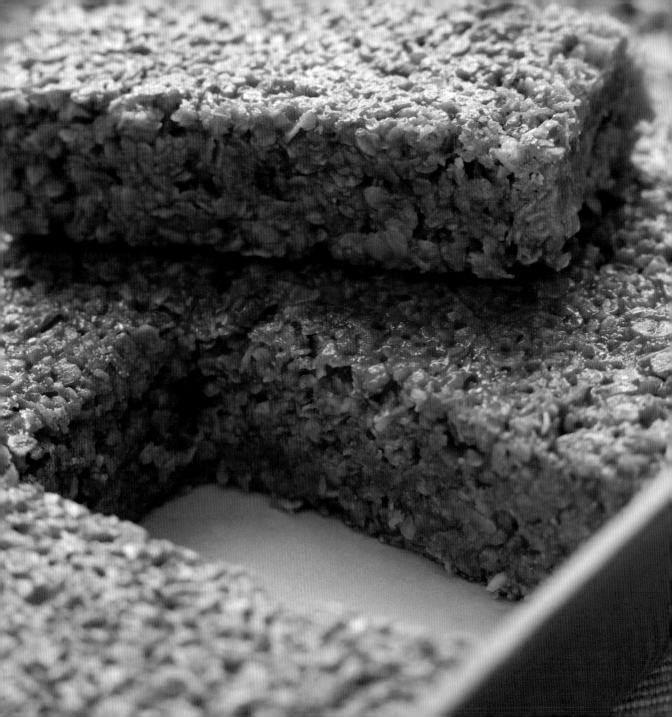

Berry Breakfast Bars

1 CUP BUCKWHEAT FLOUR
1 CUP QUINOA FLAKES
½ CUP FINELY CHOPPED, DRIED
   CRANBERRIES
¼ TEASPOON SALT
4 TEASPOONS HONEY OR AGAVE
   NECTAR
4 TEASPOONS PALM OIL SHORTENING
UP TO 1 TABLESPOON WATER OR 100%
   FRUIT JUICE

1. Preheat oven to 300°F.

2. Combine all dry ingredients, including cranberries, in a bowl. Sift with a fork until all ingredients are distributed. Add honey or agave and shortening. Stir until crumbly. While stirring, add 1–2 drops of water or juice. Keep stirring and adding liquid until a cohesive dough forms. Use your hands to mold the dough into a ball. Place the ball in a 9 x 9-inch baking pan. Press dough into the pan with the back of a spoon. Bake for no more than 10–15 minutes. Bake longer for a crispy, crunchy bar. Remove from the oven and let cool completely. Cut into bars and enjoy.

Blueberry Corn Muffins

1 CUP WHOLE GRAIN CORN FLOUR OR
   CORNMEAL
1 TEASPOON BUCKWHEAT FLOUR
   (OPTIONAL)
1 TEASPOON BAKING POWDER
   (ALUMINUM-FREE)
¼ CUP UNSWEETENED APPLESAUCE
½ CUP CORN OR CANOLA OIL
SWEETENER—¼ CUP EVAPORATED
   CANE JUICE OR AGAVE NECTAR
3–4 TEASPOONS WATER
½ CUP FROZEN BLUEBERRIES

1. Preheat oven to 400°F. Place paper liners in eight muffin pan cups.

2. Combine flours and baking powder in a medium mixing bowl. Sift thoroughly with a fork.

3. Add applesauce, oil, and sweetener. Stir with a fork until a thick batter forms.

4. Add 2 tablespoons of water at a time until batter loosens slightly.

5. Add blueberries and stir gently.

6. Spoon batter into muffin cups.

7. Bake on the middle rack of the oven for 10–15 minutes or until muffins become light brown.

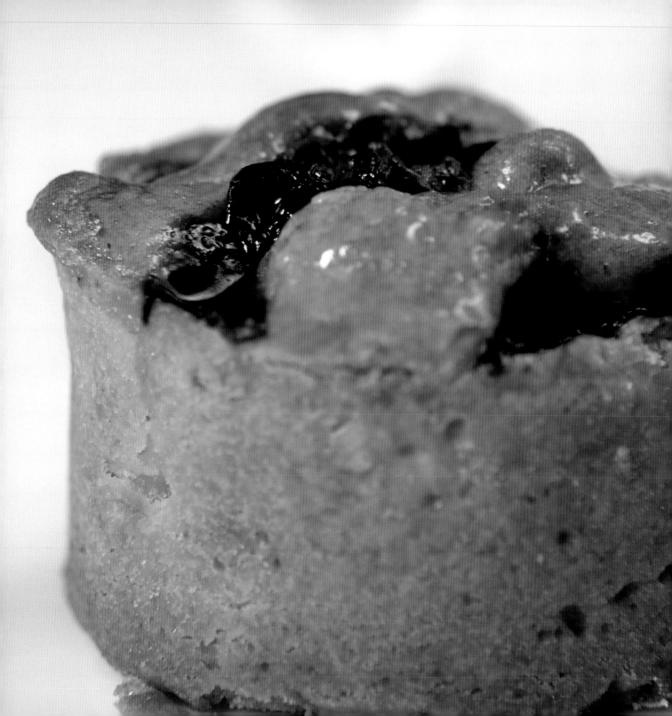

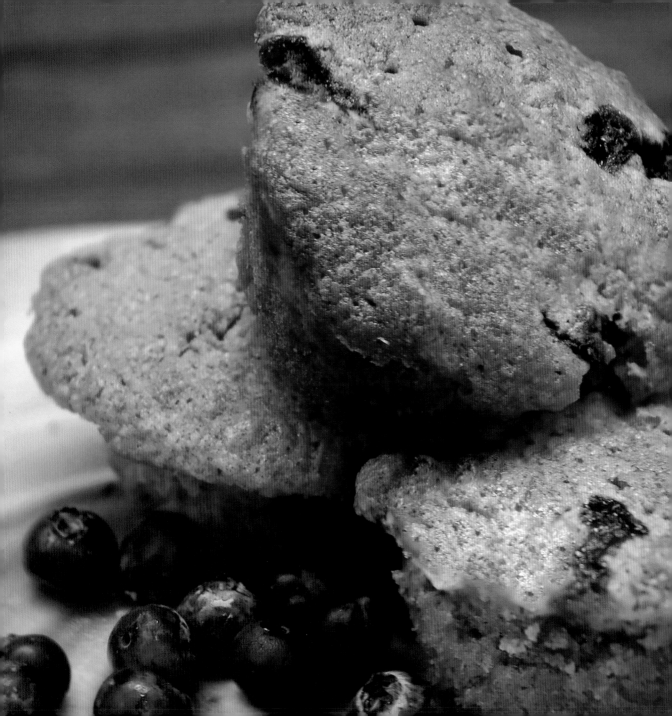

Blueberry Muffins

1 CUP BUCKWHEAT FLOUR
1 TEASPOON BAKING POWDER
   (ALUMINUM-FREE)
½ TEASPOON SALT
¾ CUP LUKEWARM WATER
¼ CUP CORN OR CANOLA OIL
SWEETENER—½ CUP EVAPORATED
   CANE JUICE OR AGAVE NECTAR
½ CUP BLUEBERRIES (IF FROZEN,
   THAW AND DRAIN EXCESS
   MOISTURE)

1. Preheat oven to 400°F. Place paper liners in eight muffin pan cups.

2. Combine flour, baking powder, and salt in a large mixing bowl. Sift thoroughly with a fork. Add water, oil, and sweetener. Mix with a large spoon until well blended.

3. Add blueberries and stir gently. Spoon batter into muffin cups. Bake on middle rack of oven until top appears brown and slightly crusty (approximately 25–30 minutes).

4. Cool completely.

Breakfast Kabobs

2   TABLESPOONS OLIVE OIL
1   MEDIUM POTATO CUBED, AND
    PEELED, IF DESIRED
1   TEASPOON EACH OF SALT, GARLIC
    POWDER, AND BLACK PEPPER
1   MEDIUM APPLE, CUBED
COOKED BREAKFAST SAUSAGE, CUT
    INTO BITE-SIZED PIECES

1. In a medium-sized bowl combine oil, potatoes,
    apple, and seasonings. Toss until well blended. Place
    potatoes and apple on a non-stick baking pan and
    bake at 400°F until potatoes and apples are soft and
    light brown. Let cool slightly. On metal skewers,
    alternate placing sausage, apple, and potato until the
    skewer is full.

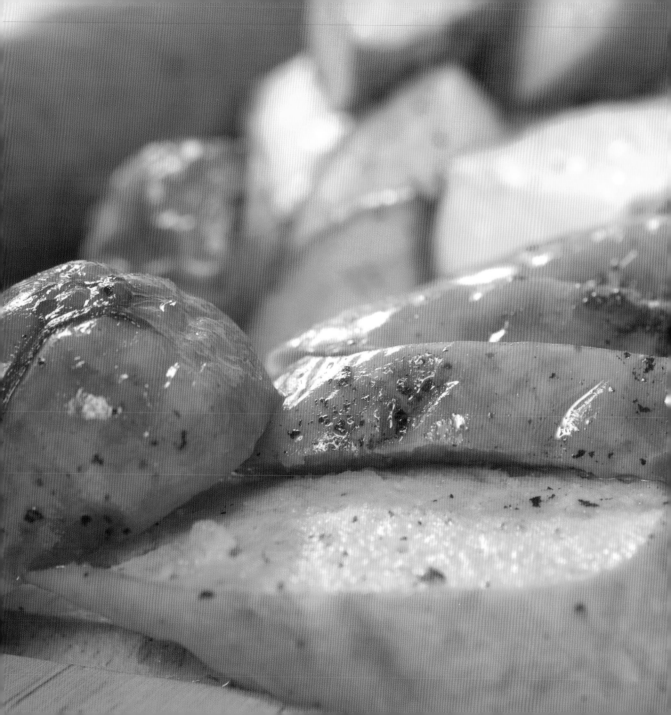

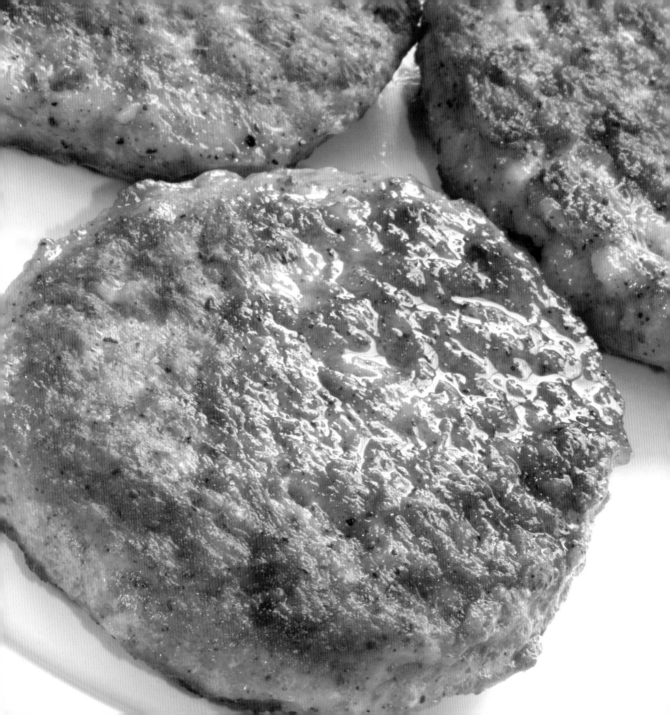

Breakfast Sausage Patties

½ LB GROUND TURKEY
1 TEASPOON EACH OF DRIED, FINELY
   GROUND SAGE LEAVES, THYME
   LEAVES, AND ROSEMARY LEAVES
1 TEASPOON ALLSPICE SEASONING
1 TEASPOON GARLIC POWDER
1 TEASPOON SALT
1 TEASPOON GROUND BLACK PEPPER
2 TABLESPOONS MOLASSES

1. Combine all ingredients in a large mixing bowl. Mix thoroughly until the meat is smooth.

2. For best flavor, cover tightly and marinate in the refrigerator for at least 2 hours.

3. Use your hands to form 2-inch round patties.

4. Heat a non-stick skillet to medium setting. Cook thoroughly on each side.

Grits with Bacon

2   CUPS CHICKEN BROTH
½   TEASPOON SALT
½   TEASPOON GROUND BLACK PEPPER
¼   TEASPOON GARLIC POWDER
1   CUP QUICK GRITS
3   SLICES OF UNCURED PORK OR
     TURKEY BACON, COOKED AND
     CHOPPED

1. Combine chicken broth, salt, pepper, and garlic powder in a small pot. Bring to a boil and stir until salt is dissolved.

2. Add grits and reduce heat to low. Stir constantly until boiling stops.

3. Cover and cook over low heat until grits start to thicken (2–5 minutes).

4. Crumble bacon over grits. Stir and serve warm.

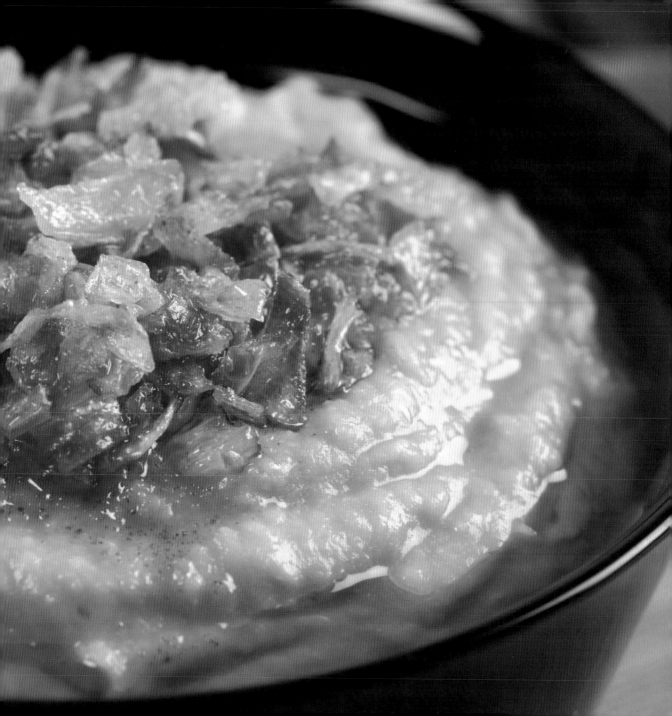

Home Fries

2   LARGE POTATOES
2   TABLESPOONS OLIVE OIL
½   CUP EACH OF CHOPPED ONION AND
     GREEN BELL PEPPER
1   TEASPOON EACH OF SALT AND
     GROUND BLACK PEPPER
¼   CUP WATER

1. Peel and cube the potatoes. Heat olive oil in a large skillet to medium setting. Add potatoes, onion, green pepper, salt, and black pepper. Sautee and stir until vegetables are soft. Stir in water and reduce heat to low setting. Cover and let simmer until potatoes are soft.

Orange Essence Cranberry Muffins

1   CUP BUCKWHEAT FLOUR
1   TEASPOON BAKING POWDER
    (ALUMINUM-FREE)
½   TEASPOON SALT
2   TABLESPOONS ORANGE PEEL,
    MINCED
½   CUP DRIED CRANBERRIES, CHOPPED
¾   CUP LUKEWARM WATER
¼   CUP CORN OR CANOLA OIL
SWEETENER—½ CUP EVAPORATED
    CANE JUICE OR AGAVE NECTAR

1. Preheat oven to 400°F. Place paper liners in muffin pan cups.

2. In a medium mixing bowl, stir together flour, baking powder, salt, orange peel, and cranberries. Stir in water, oil, and sweetener. Spoon batter into muffin cups. Bake until the tops of the muffins appear light brown and crusty (approximately 25–30 minutes).

3. Cool completely.

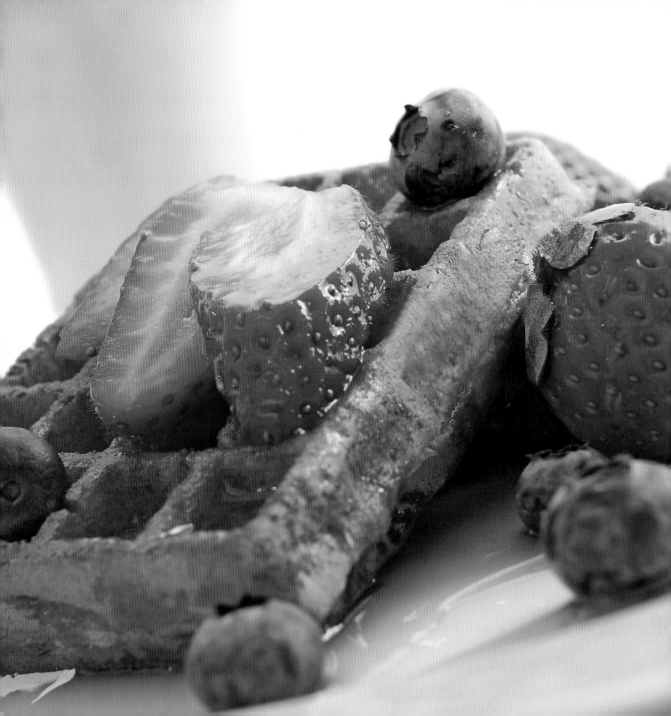

Pancakes and Waffles

1 CUP BUCKWHEAT FLOUR
2 TABLESPOONS BAKING POWDER
   (ALUMINUM-FREE)
1½ TEASPOONS SALT
¼ CUP CORN OR CANOLA OIL
2 CUPS LUKEWARM WATER
1 TABLESPOON GLUTEN-FREE
   VANILLA

1. Combine flour, baking powder, and salt in a small bowl. Sift thoroughly with a fork. Add oil, water, and vanilla. Mix well. If needed, add water by the teaspoon until batter loosens slightly.

- For pancakes, preheat non-stick griddle or frying pan to medium heat setting. Brush lightly with oil. Pour 5-inch circles of batter onto hot cooking surface. Cook on each side for approximately 2 minutes or until brown.

- For waffles, preheat waffle iron. Brush lightly with oil. Pour batter onto waffle iron. Cook until crispy, using waffle maker guidelines.

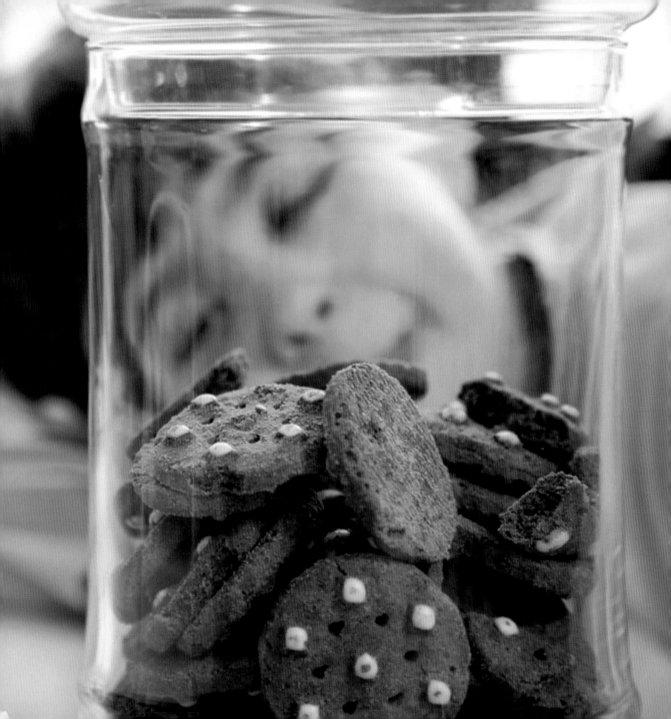

Sweet Treats

Apple Fritters

1 CUP BUCKWHEAT FLOUR
1 TABLESPOON CORNMEAL
¼ CUP EVAPORATED CANE JUICE
1 TEASPOON SALT
1 TEASPOON BAKING POWDER
1 TEASPOON GROUND CINNAMON
1 CUP WATER
¼ CUP CORN OR CANOLA OIL
OIL FOR DEEP FRYING
2 PEELED APPLES, SLICED INTO
   ¼-INCH-THICK WEDGES

1. Stir together dry ingredients in a medium bowl. Stir in water and oil. Add apple wedges and stir until wedges are covered.

2. Pick up one apple wedge at a time with metal tongs. Place apple wedges into hot oil and fry (up to six at a time) until batter appears medium brown.

3. Remove with a spatula and drain excess oil.

4. Do not over cook. Cool completely before eating.

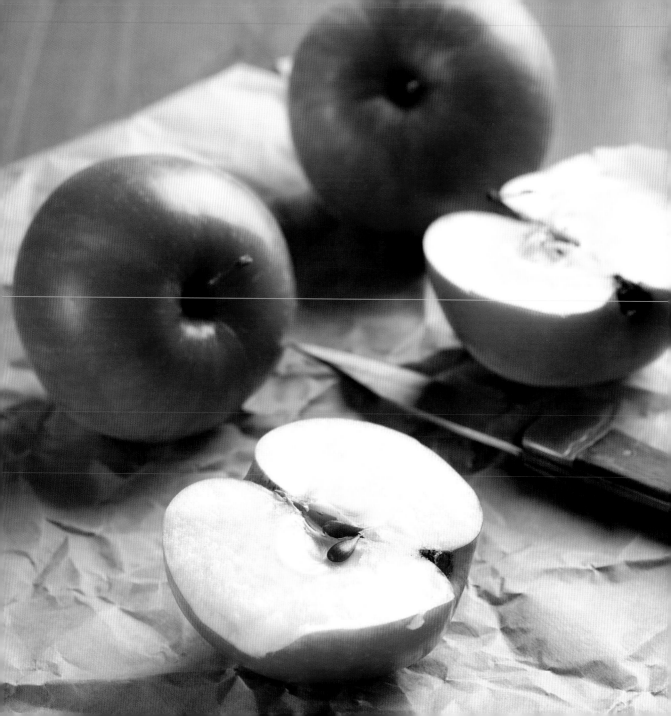

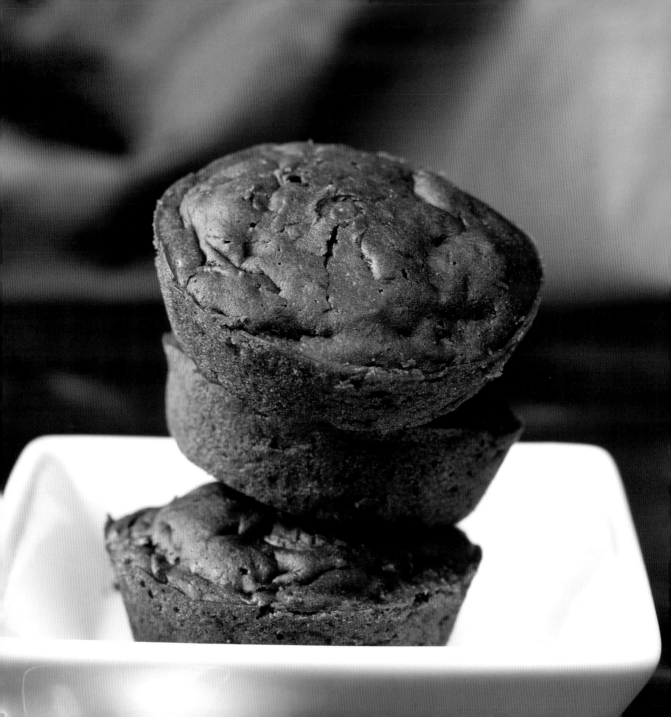

Brownie Bites

1 CUP UNSWEETENED DARK COCOA
   POWDER
1 TABLESPOON BAKING POWDER
   (ALUMINUM-FREE)
1 TEASPOON SALT
SWEETENER—1 ½ CUPS EVAPORATED
   CANE JUICE OR ¾
   CUP AGAVE NECTAR
2½ CUPS LUKEWARM WATER
½ CUP CORN OR CANOLA OIL
1 TABLESPOON GLUTEN-FREE
   VANILLA EXTRACT

1. Preheat oven to 400°F.

2. Combine flour, cocoa, baking powder, and salt in a large mixing bowl. Sift thoroughly with a fork. Set aside.

3. Add sweetener, water, oil, and vanilla. Stir with a whisk until blended.

4. Add extra water by the tablespoon if the batter is too thick to stir.

5. Pour batter into miniature muffin cups or into a 9 x 9-inch square baking dish.

6. Bake on the middle rack of the oven for approximately 20–25 minutes or until the top appears slightly crusty.

7. Remove from the oven and place pan on a cooling rack. Cool completely before removing.

Suggested topping: Lightly roast 1 cup of raw pumpkin seeds or sunflower seeds on the stovetop. Let cool slightly. Place in a blender and pulse until crumbly. Stir into batter or sprinkle on top before placing in the oven.

The Autism Cookbook

Carrot Cake

2   CUPS BUCKWHEAT FLOUR
1   TABLESPOON BAKING POWDER
    (ALUMINUM-FREE)
2   TABLESPOONS GROUND CINNAMON
1   TEASPOON GROUND NUTMEG
½   TEASPOON SALT
SWEETENER—1 CUP EVAPORATED
    CANE JUICE OR ½ CUP AGAVE
    NECTAR
1   CUP UNSWEETENED APPLESAUCE
1   CUP SHREDDED CARROTS
½   CUP RAISINS
¼   CUP LUKEWARM WATER
1   CUP CORN OR CANOLA OIL
1   TABLESPOON GLUTEN-FREE
    VANILLA EXTRACT

1. Preheat oven to 400°F.

2. Combine flour, baking powder, cinnamon, nutmeg, and salt in a large mixing bowl. Sift thoroughly with a fork.

3. Add sweetener, applesauce, carrots, raisins, water, oil, and vanilla. Mix with a large spoon until well blended.

4. Pour mixture into a non-stick, 9 ½-inch bundt pan

5. Bake on the middle rack of the oven until top appears brown and slightly crusty (approximately 40–50 minutes).

6. Cool completely. Carefully invert the pan to remove the cake.

Top with Vanilla Glaze on page 227 and serve.

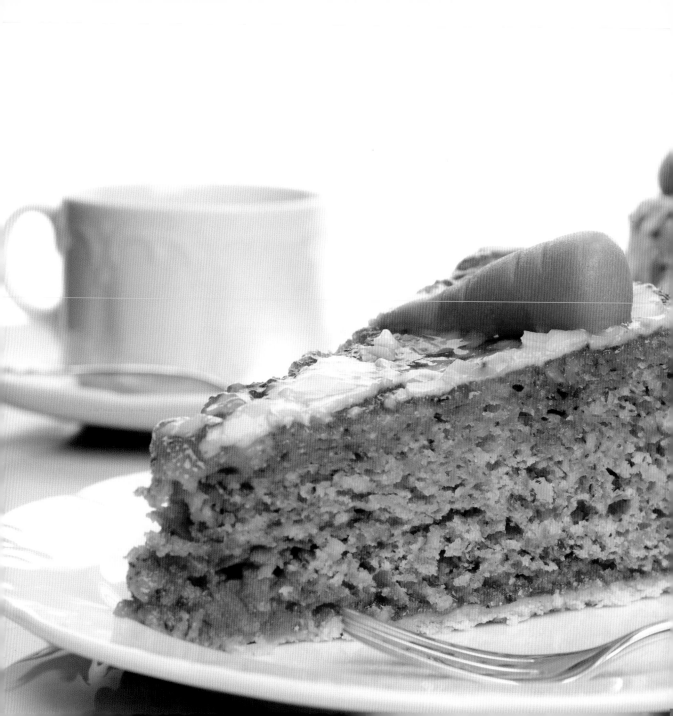

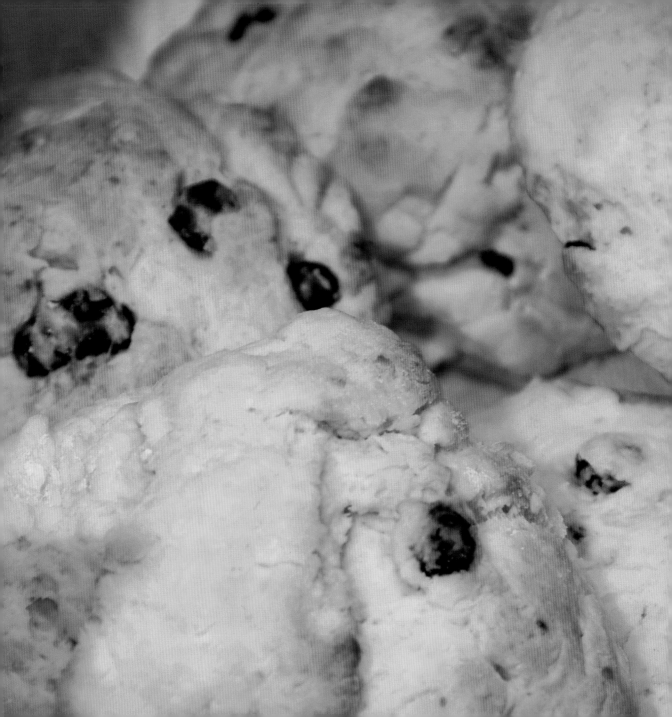

Chocolate Chip Scones

¾ CUP BUCKWHEAT FLOUR
½ CUP POTATO FLOUR
2 TEASPOONS BAKING POWDER
½ CUP PALM OIL SHORTENING
½ CUP AGAVE NECTAR
¼ CUP WATER
¼ CUP APPLE CIDER VINEGAR
½ CUP CHOCOLATE CHIPS

1. Combine dry ingredients in a bowl and sift with a fork. Add shortening, nectar, water, vinegar, and chips. Mix until a ball of dough forms. Place the dough on a flat surface and push it gently down to form a 1-inch-thick circle. Cut the dough into wedges and place each wedge on a baking sheet. Brush the top of the scones lightly with oil. Bake for 12–15 minutes or until scones are light brown.

Cinnamon-Raisin Cookies

2   CUPS BUCKWHEAT FLOUR
¼   CUP QUINOA FLAKES
½   TEASPOON SALT
1½ TEASPOONS GROUND CINNAMON
1   CUP RAISINS
½   CUP CORN OR CANOLA OIL
SWEETENER—1 CUP EVAPORATED
    CANE JUICE OR ½ CUP AGAVE
    NECTAR
UP TO ½ CUP COLD WATER IF USING
    EVAPORATED CANE JUICE

1. Preheat oven to 375°F.

2. Combine flour, quinoa flakes, salt, cinnamon, and raisins in a large mixing bowl. Sift thoroughly with a fork.

3. Add oil and sweetener. Mix with a fork until a clean ball of dough forms.

4. If using evaporated cane juice, add ¼ cup of water at a time to make the dough stick together.

5. Scoop dough with the tip of a spoon. Use your hands to form a 1-inch ball. Flatten slightly.

6. Place dough on a baking sheet three inches apart.

7. Bake on the top rack of the oven for 12–15 minutes.

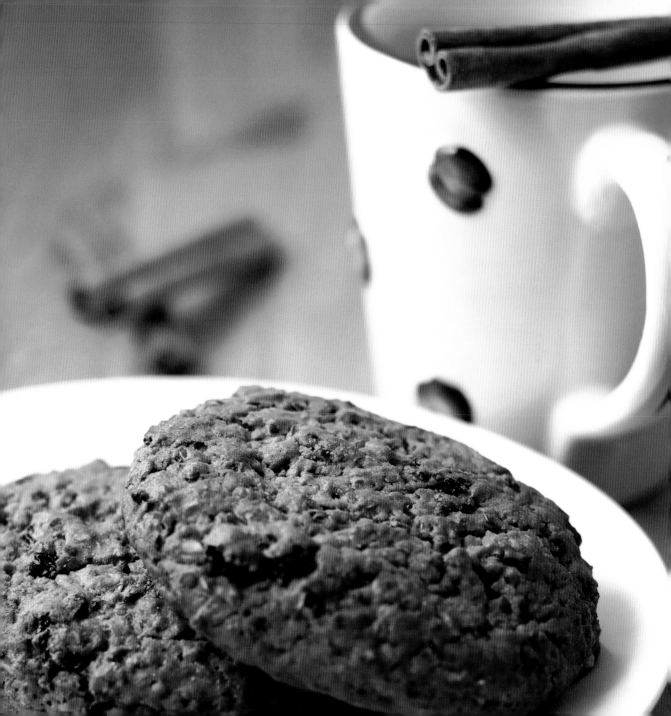

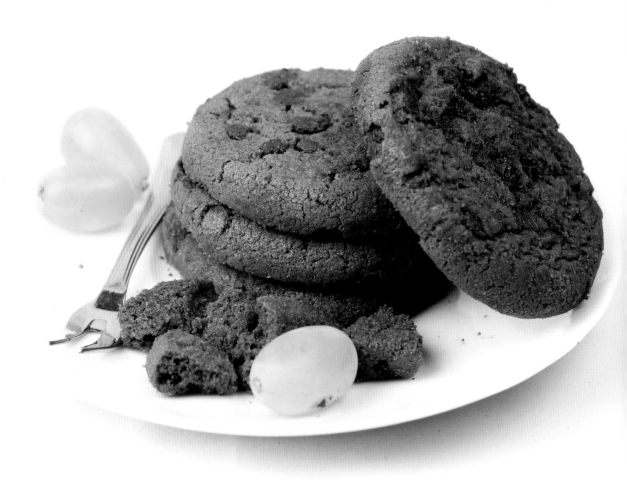

Cocoa Cookies

1 CUP BUCKWHEAT FLOUR
½ CUP UNSWEETENED DARK COCOA
  POWDER
1 TEASPOON SALT
½ CUP EVAPORATED CANE JUICE
¼ CUP CORN OR CANOLA OIL
½ CUP COLD WATER
1 TEASPOON GLUTEN-FREE VANILLA
½ CUP GFCF CHOCOLATE CHIPS
  (OPTIONAL)

1. Preheat oven to 400°F.

2. Combine flour, cocoa, and salt in a large mixing bowl. Sift thoroughly with a fork.

3. Add oil, water, vanilla, and chocolate chips. Stir until blended. The dough will be thick and sticky.

4. Scoop dough with the tip of a spoon and drop onto a baking sheet, three inches apart. Use your finger tips to gently flatten the dough and form a circle.

5. Bake on the top rack of the oven for 12–15 minutes or until cookies are slightly crusty on top.

6. Cool slightly before serving.

Coconut "Ice Cream" (Raw)

2 CUPS FRESH COCONUT, CUT INTO
    SMALL PIECES
¼ TEASPOON SALT
1 TABLESPOON GLUTEN-FREE VANILLA
    EXTRACT
CHILLED WATER OR THE MILK OF A
    FRESH COCONUT
ANY SWEETENER OF CHOICE TO TASTE

1. Combine coconut and salt in a blender and blend at high speed for 4 minutes.

2. Continue to blend. Open the lid and add vanilla extract.

3. Add water or coconut milk, ¼ cup at a time, until a thick paste forms. Turn blender off.

4. Add sweetener to taste. Stir to blend.

5. Serve cold or frozen.

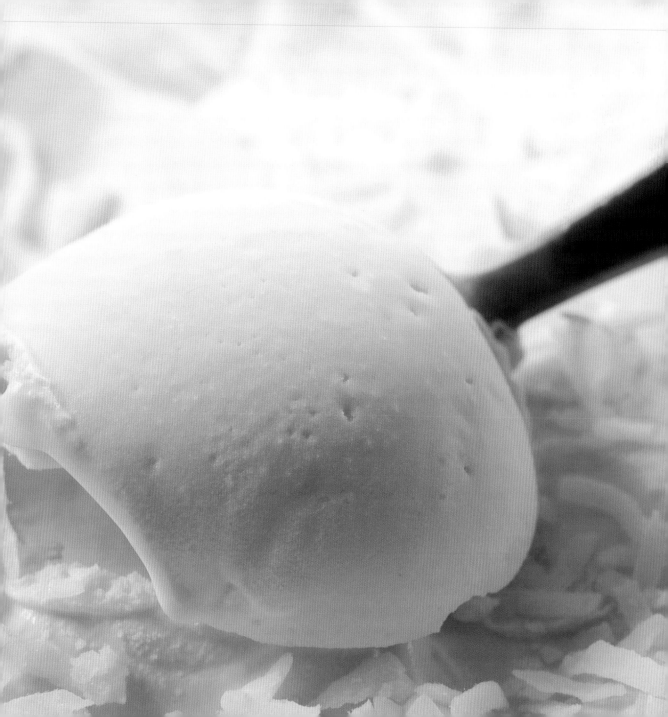

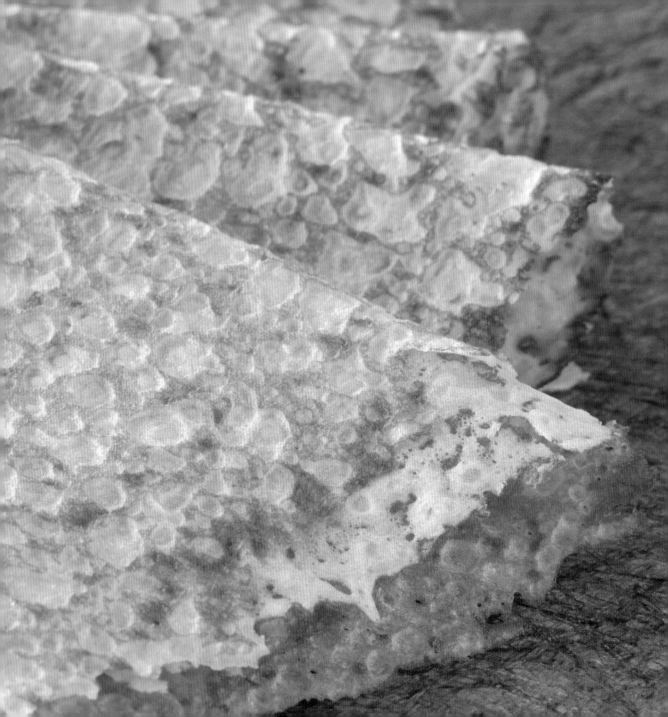

Crepes

2   CUPS WATER
¼   TEASPOON XANTHAN GUM
1   TEASPOON SALT
1   CUP BUCKWHEAT FLOUR
2   TABLESPOONS CORN OR CANOLA
    OIL

1. Combine water and salt in a medium mixing bowl. Blend with a whisk. Continue to whisk and sprinkle xanthan gum into mixture. Add ¼ cup of flour and mix well. Add ¼ cup of oil and mix well. Continue to alternate between flour and oil until everything is added. Brush oil lightly on to a 6- to 8-inch, non-stick skillet. Set the skillet over medium-high heat. Pour ¼ cup of batter onto the skillet and immediately tilt the skillet in each direction so the batter will spread. Use a spatula to lift the crepe and turn it over. Cook for a few seconds until the batter sticks together. Remove and place on a plate to cool slightly. Fill the crepe with your favorite fillings and fold or roll up.

Serving suggestions:

- Fill with strawberries or other fruit marinated in agave nectar. Fold in half and drizzle strawberry sauce over the top. Garnish with powdered sugar.
- Fill and top with chocolate glaze on page 227. Serve with fresh fruit.
- Fill with cooked breakfast sausage and home fries. Roll up and garnish with chives.
- Use as a soft tortilla shell for tacos or enchiladas on page 45.
- Roll up and dip into sesame butter recipe or avocado spread on page 221.
- Use as a sandwich roll. Fill with sliced deli meat, shredded lettuce, oil, vinegar, and oregano.

Crispy Cereal Treats

6 CUPS PUFFED CORN CEREAL
4 CUPS MINIATURE MARSHMALLOWS
½ CUP CORN OR CANOLA OIL

1. Place cereal in a blender and pulse until crumbly. Pour into a large bowl and set aside.

2. Combine marshmallows and oil in a medium saucepan. Over very low heat, melt marshmallows, stirring constantly.

3. Pour marshmallows into a cereal bowl. Stir with a large fork until marshmallows are evenly distributed.

4. Press mixture tightly into a 9-inch, square baking dish. Pack as tightly as possible. This may result in some extra space in the pan.

5. Place the dish on a cooling rack. Let cool slightly; cut into 3-inch squares.

6. Serve slightly warm.

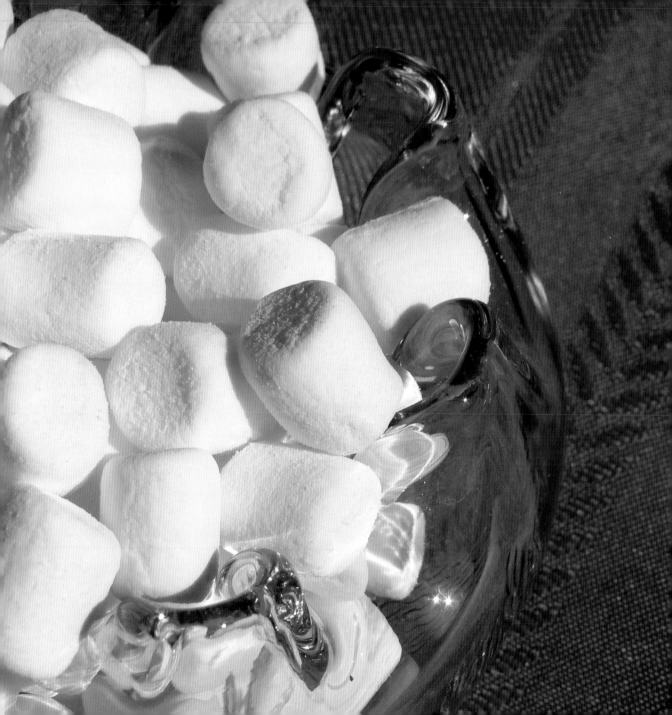

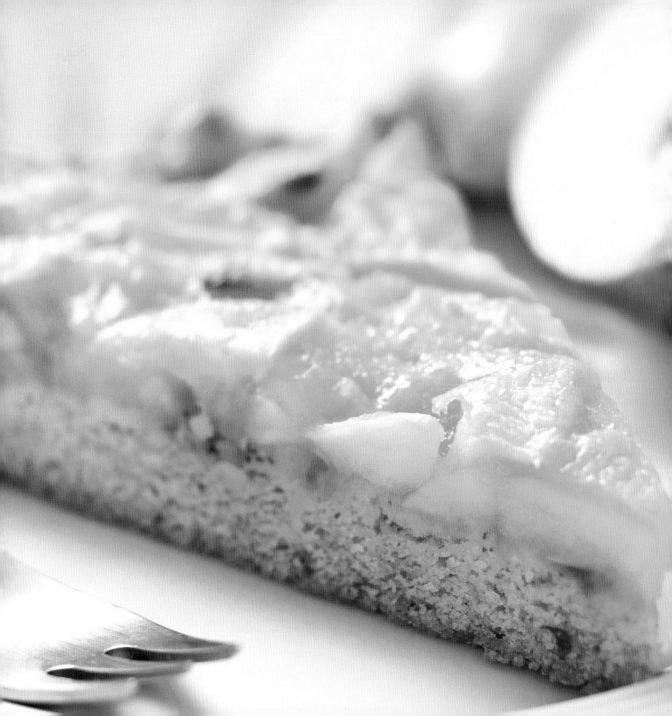

Crusty Apple Cake

CRUSTING:
- 2 CUPS LIGHTLY ROASTED PUMPKIN SEEDS OR SUNFLOWER SEEDS
- ¼ CUP FLAX SEED MEAL
- 1 TEASPOON SALT
- ½ CUP DARK BROWN SUGAR

TOPPING:
- 2 LARGE APPLES, PEELED AND SLICED

CAKE
- 2 CUPS BUCKWHEAT FLOUR
- 1 TABLESPOON BAKING POWDER
- 1 TEASPOON GROUND CINNAMON
- 1 CUP AGAVE NECTAR OR EVAPORATED CANE JUICE
- 1½ CUPS WATER
- 1 CUP CORN OR CANOLA OIL
- 2 LARGE APPLES, PEELED AND SLICED

1. In a blender, combine seeds and salt. Blend on high speed until flaky. Pour into a bowl and mix in brown sugar. Spread evenly onto the bottom of a 9-inch baking pan. Set aside.

2. In a large mixing bowl, combine dry ingredients. Sift with a fork until well blended. Add wet ingredients and stir until a smooth batter forms. Pour batter over the crusting. Carefully place apples over the batter. Bake for 45 minutes or until the cake is light brown and firm to the touch.

Deep-Dish Apple or Peach Crisp

2 LARGE GALA APPLES OR PEACHES,
   PEELED AND SLICED
¼ CUP RAISINS
SWEETENER—½ CUP EVAPORATED
   CANE JUICE OR AGAVE NECTAR
1 TEASPOON GROUND CINNAMON
½ TEASPOON SALT
1 TABLESPOON CORN OR CANOLA OIL
1 TEASPOON GLUTEN-FREE VANILLA
   EXTRACT

CRUMB TOPPING
1 CUP QUINOA OR BUCKWHEAT FLOUR
½ CUP LIGHT BROWN SUGAR, LOOSELY
   PACKED
½ TEASPOON SALT
½ CUP PALM OIL SHORTENING
(OPTIONAL: USE SHORTBREAD COOKIE
   DOUGH RECIPE FOR BOTTOM CRUST)

1. Preheat oven to 350°F.

2. Combine filling ingredients in a bowl. Stir until blended. Pour into a 9-inch baking dish and set aside.

3. Prepare topping. Combine flour, brown sugar, cinnamon, and salt in a medium bowl. Sift with a fork until light and flaky. Use your fingers to sprinkle topping generously over apples.

4. Bake for 45–60 minutes, until topping is light brown.

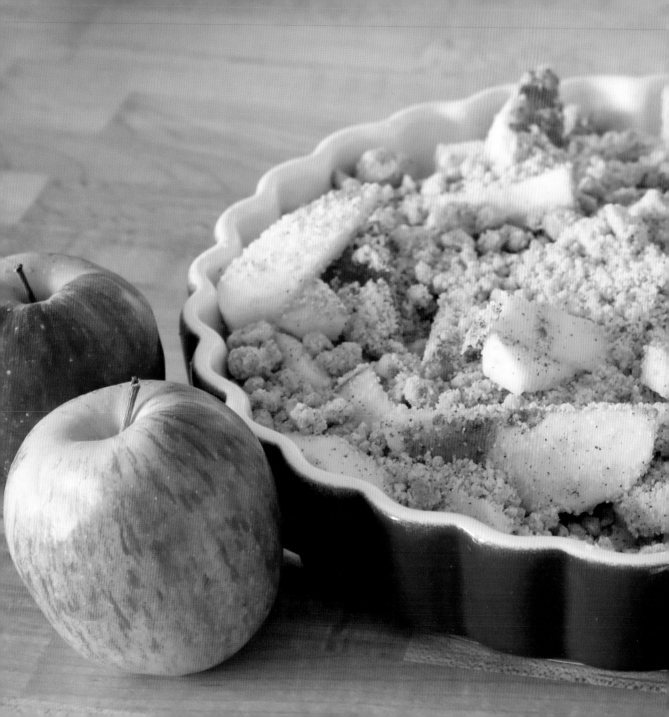

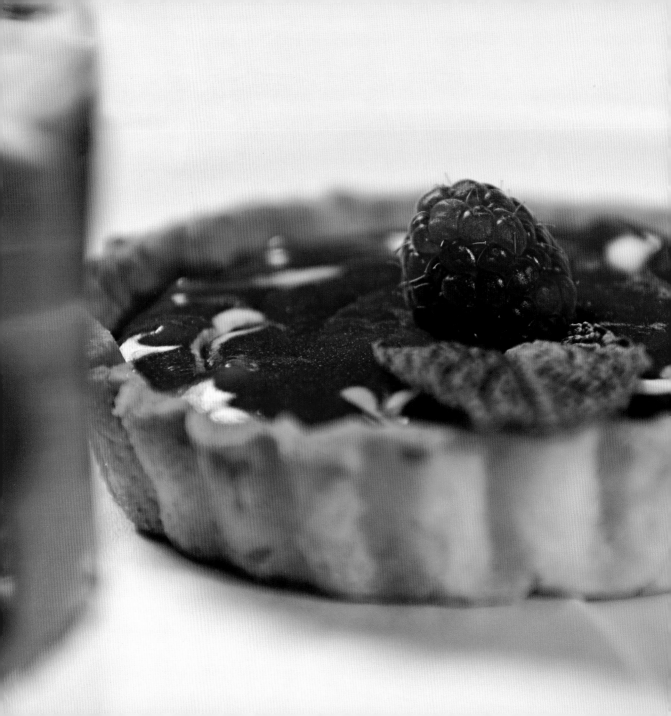

Fresh Fruit Tarts

1 SHORTBREAD COOKIE DOUGH
   RECIPE FROM PAGE 192

FILLING
1½ CUPS OF FRESH BERRIES
¼ CUP FRESH MINT LEAVES, CHOPPED
SWEETENER—2 TABLESPOONS
   EVAPORATED CANE JUICE OR AGAVE
   NECTAR
½ TEASPOON SALT
1 TABLESPOON CORN OR CANOLA OIL
JUICE FROM 1 SMALL LEMON

Prepare outer shell:

1. Preheat oven to 400°F.

2. Prepare one batch of Shortbread Cookie dough recipe.

3. Use your hands to mold the dough into individual tart or quiche baking cups. Use a knife to trim excess dough.

4. Bake tarts for 30 minutes or until brown. Set aside and let cool.

Prepare fruit filling:

5. In a large bowl, combine and stir berries, mint leaves, sweetener, salt, oil, and lemon juice.

6. Heat a non-stick skillet on low setting. Add fruit and toss gently for 2 minutes.

7. Remove from the heat and pour fruit into tart cups.

8. Serve slightly warm.

Fruit Sorbet (Raw)

FRESH FRUIT,
IF USING:
BLUEBERRIES: 2 CUPS
STRAWBERRIES: 2 CUPS
PEELED MANGO: 2 CUPS
RASPBERRIES: 3 CUPS
CHOICE OF SWEETENER—½ CUP AGAVE
    NECTAR OR ½ CUP HONEY

1. Place all ingredients in a blender.

2. Puree at high speed until mixture becomes smooth.

3. Pour contents into freezer-safe container. Cover and freeze.

4. Serve frozen. Use ice cream scoop to serve.

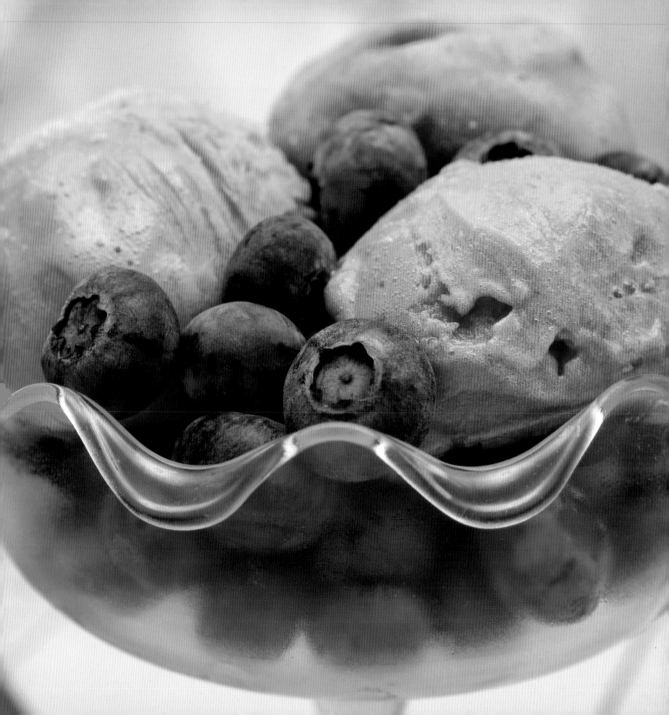

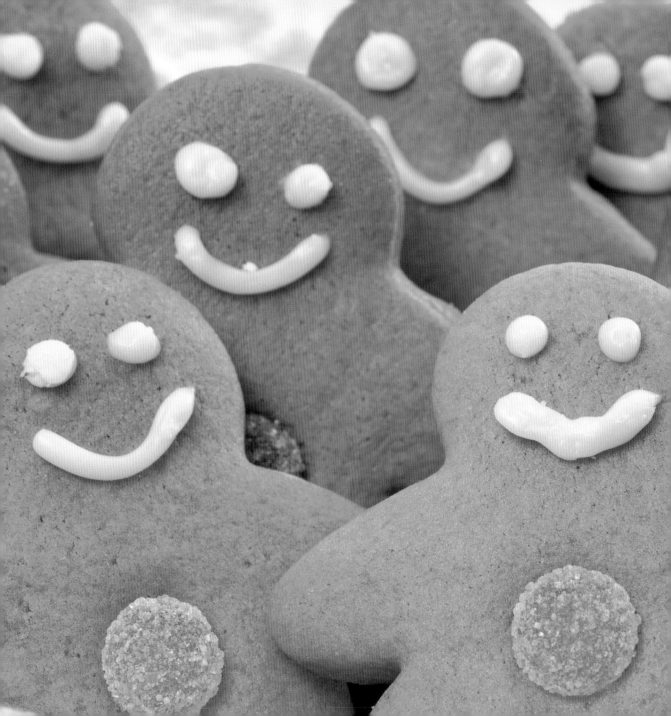

Gingerbread Cookies

2 CUPS BUCKWHEAT FLOUR
½ TEASPOON SALT
½ TEASPOON GROUND GINGER
   POWDER
½ TEASPOON ALLSPICE SEASONING
½ CUP CORN OR CANOLA OIL
2 TABLESPOONS MOLASSES
SWEETENER — 1 CUP EVAPORATED
   CANE JUICE OR ½ CUP AGAVE
   NECTAR
½ CUP COLD WATER IF USING
   EVAPORATED CANE JUICE

1. Preheat oven to 375°F.

2. In a large bowl, combine flour, salt, ginger powder, and allspice. Sift with a fork until well blended.

3. Add oil, molasses, and sweetener.

4. If using evaporated cane juice, add water by the tablespoon and stir until a clean ball of dough forms.

5. Separate dough to make five smaller balls of dough. Flatten each ball with your hands over a clean, flat surface.

6. Use a small cookie cutter to cut dough into the shape of a person. Use a butter knife to scrape excess surrounding dough (collect to create another ball). Continue until all the dough is used.

7. Use a spatula to scoop dough and place on a non-stick cookie sheet.

8. Bake approximately 15 minutes. Cool completely.

9. To decorate, use vanilla-flavored frosting on page 228. Place frosting in a small zipper-seal sandwich bag. Cut a ¼-inch hole on the bottom edge of the frosting bag. Squeeze frosting out to decorate.

Old-Fashioned Shortbread Cookies

2 CUPS BUCKWHEAT FLOUR
½ TEASPOON SALT
½ CUP PALM OIL SHORTENING
1 TEASPOON GLUTEN-FREE VANILLA
   EXTRACT
½ CUP EVAPORATED CANE JUICE OR
   AGAVE NECTAR
UP TO ½ CUP WATER IF USING
   EVAPORATED CANE JUICE

1. Combine flour and salt in a medium mixing bowl. Stir until blended. Stir in shortening, vanilla, and sweetener. If using evaporated cane juice as a sweetener, add water by the tablespoon until dough sticks together. Form 1-inch balls of dough with your hands. Place dough on a non-stick baking sheet, 2 inches apart. Flatten the dough with your finger tips to form a circle. Bake for 10–12 minutes. Use a spatula to remove the cookies from the baking sheet while still hot. Cool completely before serving.

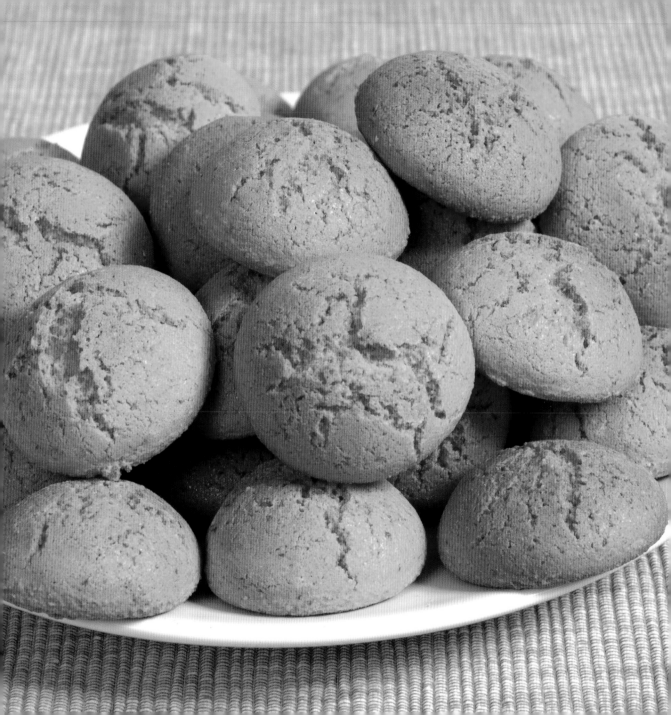

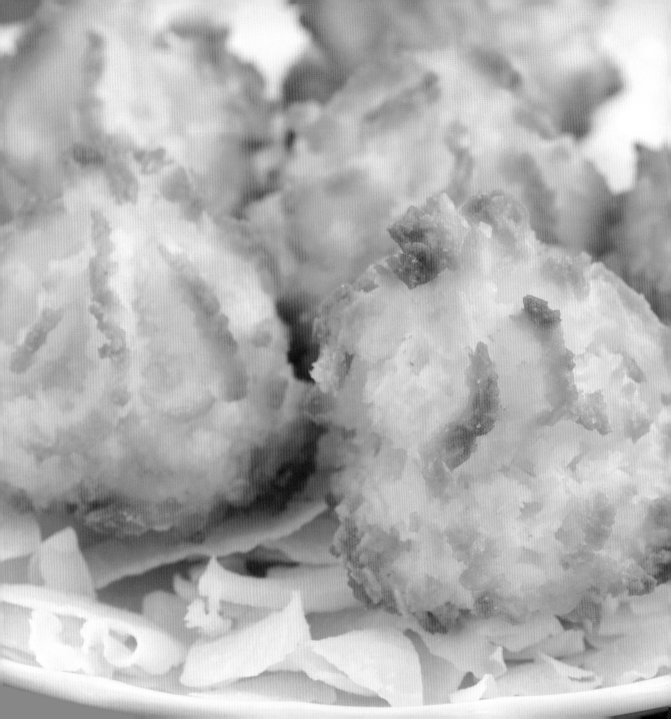

Perfect Macaroons

1½ CUPS WATER

SWEETENER—1 CUP AGAVE NECTAR OR
EVAPORATED CANE JUICE

2 TEASPOONS GLUTEN-FREE VANILLA
EXTRACT

½ TEASPOON SALT

½ CUP BUCKWHEAT FLOUR OR QUINOA
FLOUR

3 CUPS FINELY SHREDDED COCONUT
(UNSWEETENED)

1. Preheat oven to 375°F. In a medium mixing bowl, combine water, sweetener, vanilla, and salt and stir with a whisk until blended. Add flour and coconut. Stir with a spoon until blended. Drop batter by the tablespoon onto a non-stick baking sheet, 2 inches apart. Bake for 15 minutes or until macaroons appear light brown.

Rocky Trail Mix Bars

1½ CUPS BUCKWHEAT FLOUR

¾ CUP EVAPORATED CANE JUICE

½ TEASPOON SALT

¼ TEASPOON CARDAMOM

¼ CUP EACH OF PUMPKIN SEEDS,
RAISINS, AND DRIED MANGO,
COARSELY CHOPPED IN A FOOD
PROCESSOR

¼ CUP SHREDDED COCONUT

½ CUP CORN OR CANOLA OIL

½ CUP WATER

1. Combine four, cane juice, salt, cardamom, seeds, and fruit in a large mixing bowl. Sift until blended. Add oil and water. Stir until the dough sticks together. Spread the dough in a 9-inch square baking pan and bake 30–40 minutes, until light brown. Cool slightly and cut into rectangles. Cool completely before serving.

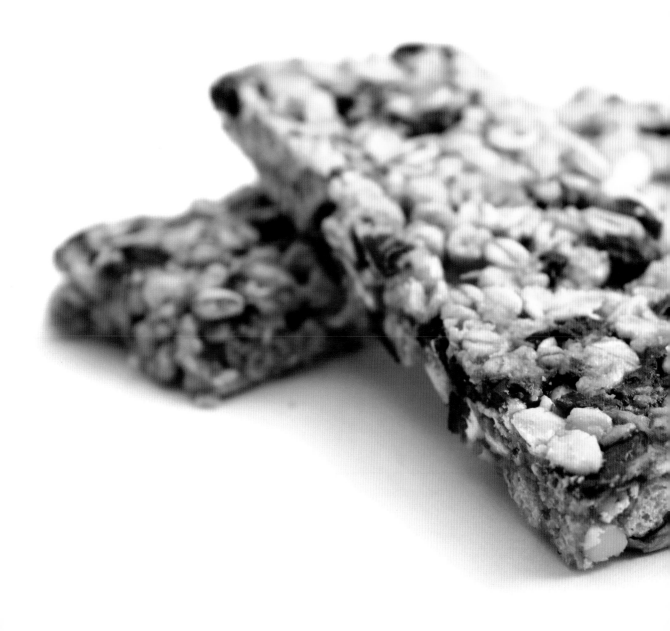

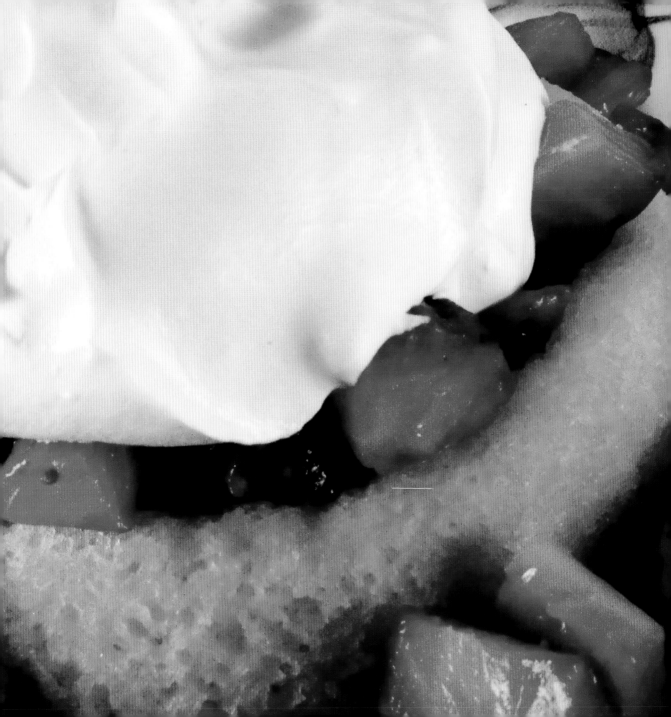

Strawberry Shortcake

5   LARGE STRAWBERRIES, SLICED
1   CORN BREAD RECIPE FROM PAGE
    129
1   VANILLA FROSTING RECIPE FROM
    PAGE 228

1. Soak strawberry slices in agave nectar, if desired. Set aside.

2. Bake Corn Bread recipe in muffin cups. Fill muffin cups only halfway to create a flat surface.

3. Remove muffins from pan and cool completely.

4. Top with strawberries and vanilla frosting.

Sweet Potato Pie

CRUST
1 RECIPE OF OLD-FASHIONED
   SHORTBREAD COOKIES ON PAGE 192

FILLING
2 FULLY COOKED SWEET POTATOES,
   COARSELY MASHED
¼ CUP BUCKWHEAT FLOUR
1 TABLESPOON GROUND CINNAMON
1 TEASPOON SALT
½ CUP EVAPORATED CANE JUICE OR
   AGAVE NECTAR
1 TEASPOON GLUTEN-FREE VANILLA
   EXTRACT
2 TABLESPOONS CORN OR CANOLA
   OIL
¼ CUP WATER

1. Preheat oven to 400°F.

2. Prepare cookie dough recipe. Use your fingertips to mold the dough along the bottom and sides of a 9-inch pie pan. Set aside.

3. Prepare filling: Place all ingredients in a large mixing bowl and stir just enough to blend everything together. Mix with an electric mixer on medium speed until smooth. Use a rubber scraper to scrape sides of the bowl often. Set aside.

4. Place the dough along the bottom and sides of a 9-inch baking pan. Use a knife to cut off any excess dough from the sides of the pan. Pour filling over the crust. Bake for 40–45 minutes. Crust should be flaky and filling should appear lightly browned. Cool completely before serving.

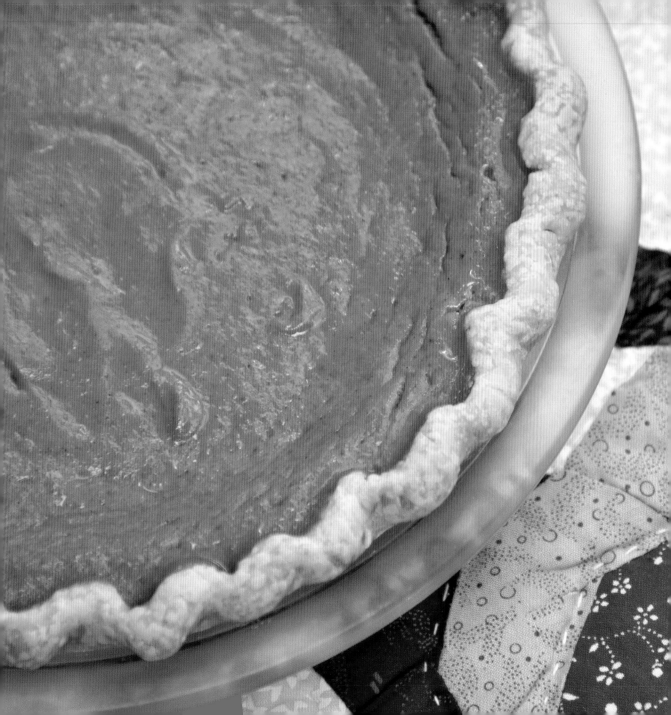

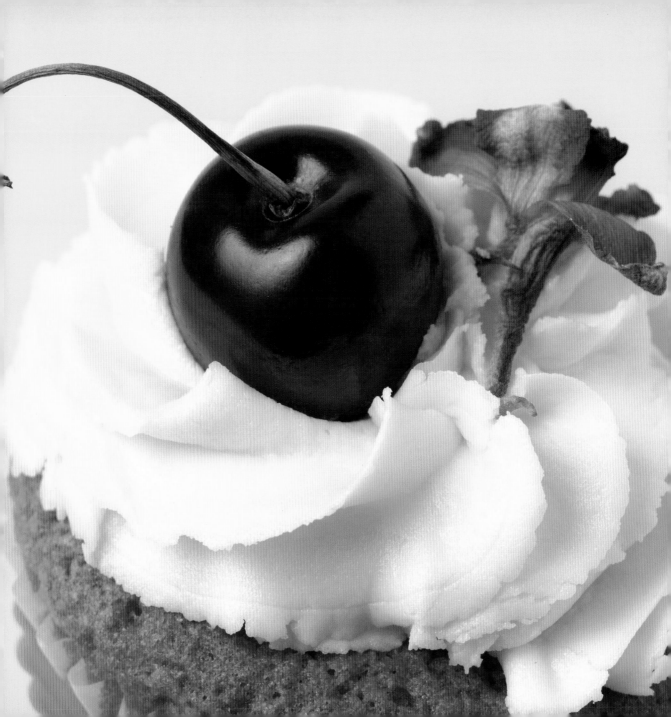

Vanilla Cupcakes

2   CUPS BUCKWHEAT FLOUR
1   TABLESPOON BAKING POWDER
    (ALUMINUM-FREE)
¼   TEASPOON SALT
1½ CUPS CORN OR CANOLA OIL
1½ CUPS WATER
SWEETENER— 1 CUP EVAPORATED
    CANE JUICE OR AGAVE NECTAR
1   TEASPOON GLUTEN-FREE VANILLA
    EXTRACT

1. Preheat oven to 400°F. Line a muffin pan with paper cup liners. Set aside.

2. In a large mixing bowl, combine flour, baking powder, and salt. Sift with a fork until well blended.

3. Add oil, water, sweetener, and vanilla. Stir until well blended.

4. Use a spoon to fill muffin cups.

5. Bake approximately 25 minutes or until cupcakes appear light brown.

Serve with Flavored Frosting on page 228.

Velvet Pudding (Raw)

2 CUPS BUCKWHEAT FLOUR
1 TABLESPOON BAKING POWDER
   (ALUMINUM-FREE)
¼ TEASPOON SALT
1½ CUPS CORN OR CANOLA OIL
1½ CUPS WATER
SWEETENER—1 CUP EVAPORATED
   CANE JUICE OR AGAVE NECTAR
1 TEASPOON GLUTEN-FREE VANILLA
   EXTRACT

1. Preheat oven to 400°F. Line a muffin pan with paper cup liners. Set aside.

2. In a large mixing bowl, combine flour, baking powder, and salt. Sift with a fork until well blended.

3. Add oil, water, sweetener, and vanilla. Stir until well blended.

4. Use a spoon to fill muffin cups.

5. Bake for approximately 25 minutes or until cupcakes appear light brown.

Serve with Flavored Frosting on page 228.

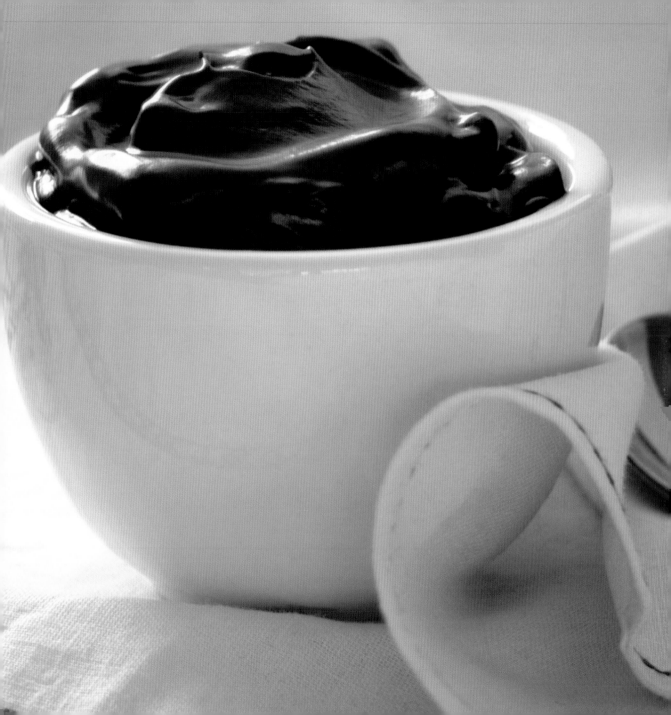

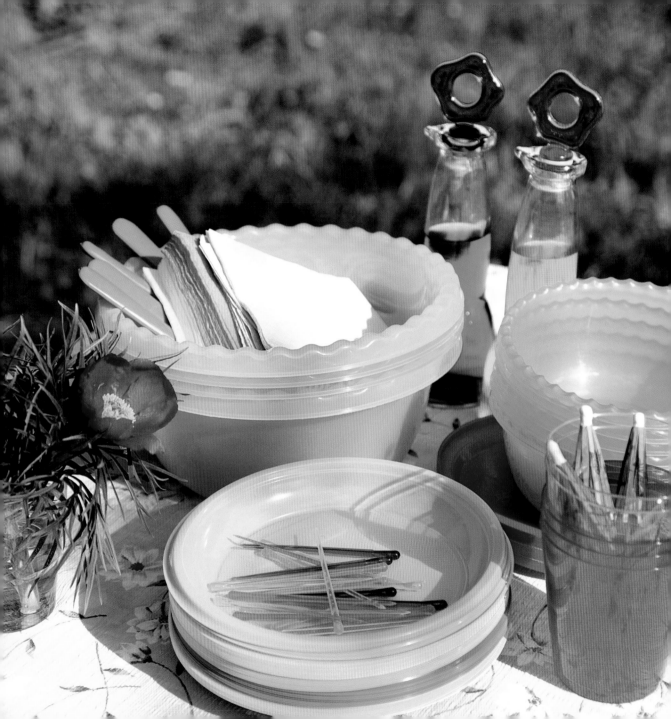

Fun Snacks

Chili Boat

5   SMALL RED POTATOES (TO MAKE
    2-INCH CIRCULAR SLICES)
½   TEASPOON OF SALT
1   TABLESPOON OLIVE OIL
2   CUPS CHILI (FROM RECIPE ON PAGE
    13)
CHOPPED CILANTRO AND SCALLION,
    SLICED INTO CIRCLES (OPTIONAL
    FOR GARNISH)

1. Wash and pat dry the potatoes. Slice the potatoes to make circles. Place the potatoes in a medium mixing bowl, add oil and salt, and stir until blended. Place the potato slices one-by-one on a non-stick baking sheet. Bake for 30–40 minutes until potatoes are soft. Let cool completely. Scoop a teaspoon of warm chili and place on top of the potatoes. Garnish with chopped cilantro and sliced scallion.

Cucumber Floaties

1   SMALL CHICKEN BREAST, COOKED
    AND CUT INTO CUBES
¼   CUP CHOPPED ONION
1   TEASPOON SALT
¼   CUP OLIVE OIL
2   TABLESPOONS WATER

1. Slice a large cucumber into circles (peel first if desired). Set aside. In a blender, combine the chicken, onion, salt, oil, and water.

2. Blend at high speed until the mixture is smooth. Add more water by the tablespoon if needed. Scoop a small amount of chicken and place it on the top of a cucumber slice. Garnish the top with chopped cilantro, minced red bell pepper, or thinly-sliced carrots for a fun color.

Sailing Banana (Raw)

LIGHTLY ROASTED PUMPKIN SEEDS OR
    SUNFLOWER SEEDS
1 SLICE OF APPLE
LARGE BANANA
RAISINS
COCONUT FLAKES (OPTIONAL)

1. Grind the seeds in a blender until flaky. Set aside. Use a knife to make small triangles (for the sail). Peel and slice a large banana into circles. Top with a raisin and coconut flakes. Carefully place the apple in the middle of the banana slice to resemble a sail.

Sesame Submarine

3   100% CORN CAKES
½ CUP SESAME BUTTER (FROM RECIPE
    ON PAGE 221)
FRESH BLUEBERRIES
FRESH STRAWBERRIES, CHOPPED

1. Cut corn cakes into fourths to make wedges.

2. Drop 1 tablespoon of sesame butter on the middle of the wedge. Top with fresh fruit.

Essential Fondue
(Fun, Nutritious, Raw)

1 CUP RAW CACAO POWDER
1 CUP RAW AGAVE NECTAR
1 TABLESPOON RAW COCONUT OIL
¼ TEASPOON SEA SALT (OPTIONAL)
FRESH STRAWBERRIES AND BANANAS
    FOR DIPPING

1. Combine cacao powder, agave, oil, and salt in a small bowl. Mix thoroughly until smooth. Use as a dip for fresh fruit. Enjoy!

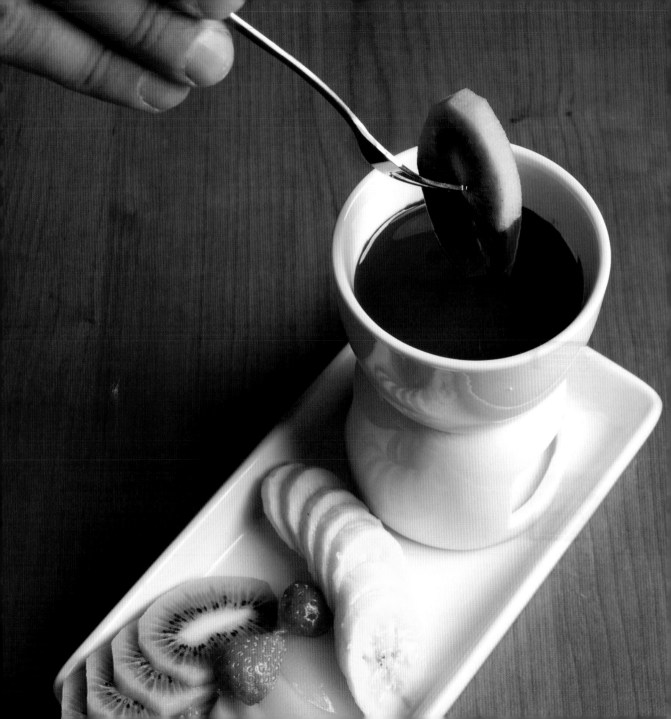

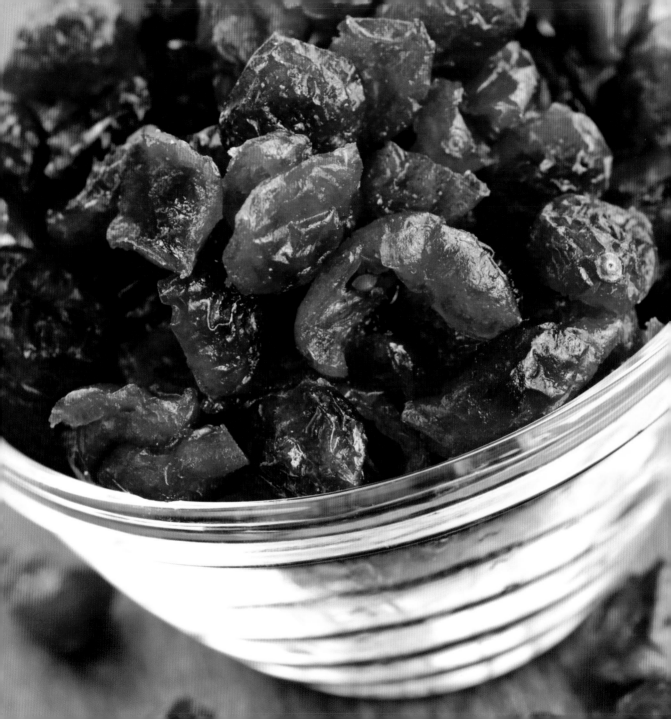

Trail Mix (Raw)

½ CUP FRESH COCONUT, DRIED AND
   SHREDDED
½ CUP EACH OF DRIED CRANBERRIES
   AND RAISINS
1 CUP RAW PUMPKIN SEEDS
1 CUP RAW SUNFLOWER SEEDS
1 TABLESPOON OIL
1 TEASPOON SALT

1. Combine all ingredients in a bowl.

2. Toss until blended.

3. Enjoy!

For a non-raw alternative, heat ingredients in a non-stick pan over low heat. Toss constantly until lightly toasted.

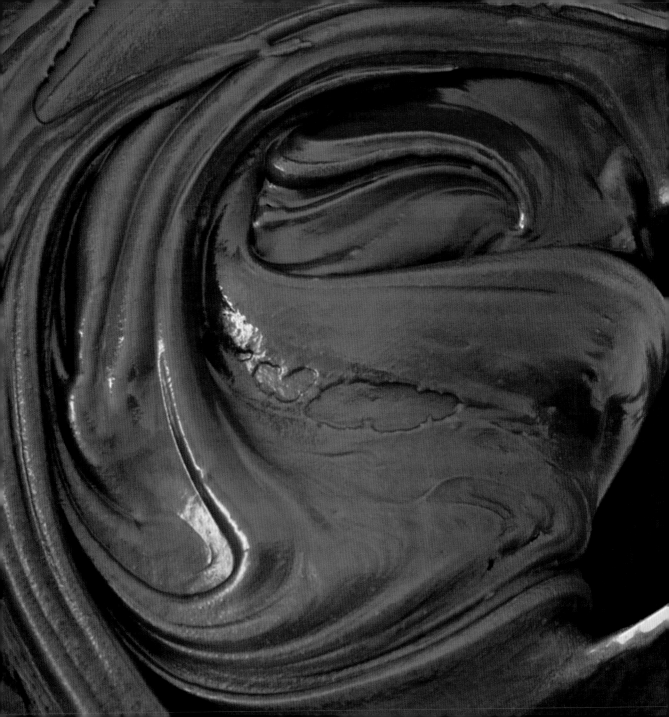

Toppings, Glazes, and Sauces

Balsamic Fusion (Raw)

3 SMALL GARLIC CLOVES, MINCED
3 FRESH BASIL LEAVES, CHOPPED
¼ CUP RAW AGAVE NECTAR
1½ TEASPOONS SEA SALT
½ TEASPOON GROUND BLACK PEPPER
½ CUP BALSAMIC VINEGAR
JUICE OF 1 LARGE LEMON
COLD-PRESSED OLIVE OIL

1. Combine garlic, basil, agave, salt, black pepper, vinegar, and lemon juice in a small bowl. Stir with a whisk until blended.

2. Continue to stir while slowly adding olive oil. Taste frequently to test. Salad dressing should be equally sweet and sour.

Serving suggestion: Toss into salad. Use romaine lettuce, cucumbers, green peppers, dried cranberries, Mandarin oranges, and uncured bacon bits.

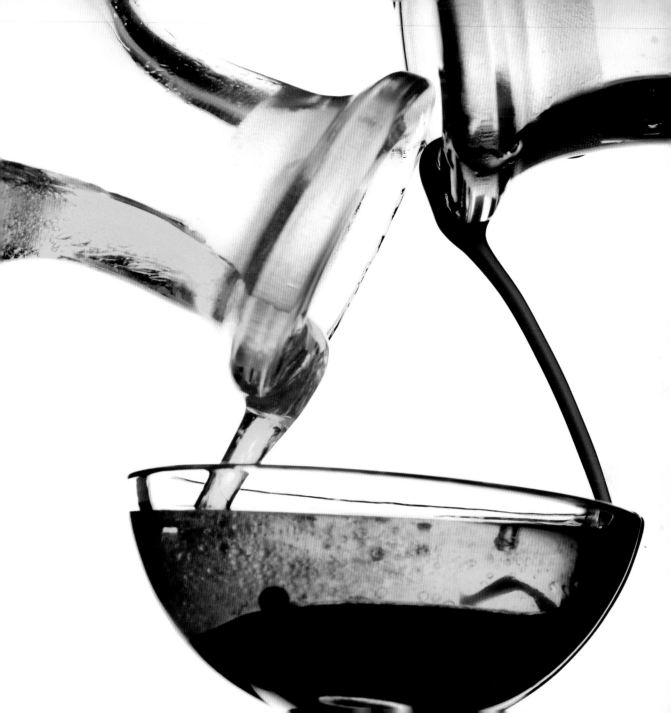

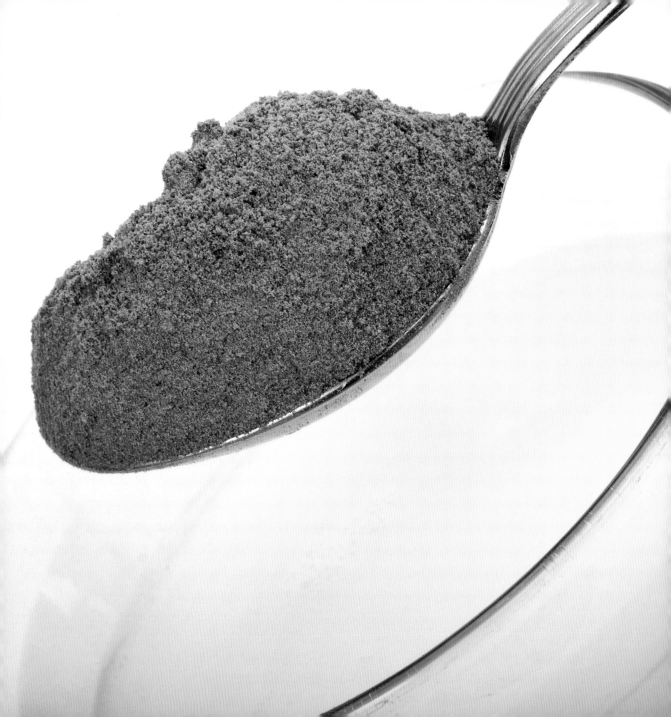

Barbecue Sauce

1   CUP HONEY
½   CUP TOMATO SAUCE
1   CUP BROWN SUGAR
2   MINCED GARLIC CLOVES
½   TEASPOON SALT
½   TEASPOON FINELY GROUND BLACK
    PEPPER
½   TEASPOON PAPRIKA

1. Combine all ingredients in a bowl. Stir well with a wire wisk. Store in a covered dish or in a bottle with a lid and refrigerate until ready to use.

Fried Onion Topping

1   DICED ONION
¼   CUP CORN MEAL
½   TEASPOON SALT (OPTIONAL)
OIL FOR DEEP FRYING

1. Heat oil in a deep fryer. In a medium mixing bowl, combine diced onion, cornmeal, and salt. Toss until onion is covered in cornmeal. Using a slotted spatula, scoop up some of the mixture, allowing excess cornmeal to drop back into the bowl. Place in hot oil and fry until light brown. Cool completely. Crumble with your fingertips and serve over mashed potatoes.

Chicken or Beef Gravy

1   CUP CHICKEN OR BEEF BROTH
    (ROOM TEMPERATURE)
¼   CUP POTATO FLOUR OR BUCKWHEAT
    FLOUR
2   TABLESPOONS CORN OR CANOLA
    OIL
2   TABLESPOONS ONION, CHOPPED
SALT AND BLACK PEPPER TO TASTE

1. Combine broth and flour in a large measuring cup.

2. Stir with a whisk until flour is dissolved. Set aside.

3. Use a small saucepan to heat oil over medium setting.

4. Add onions and sauté until slightly brown. Reduce heat to low.

5. Whisk broth/flour mixture to blend any settled flour.

6. Slowly pour broth/flour mixture into a saucepan. Stir constantly with a whisk.

7. Gravy will thicken. Remove from heat when desired thickness has been reached.

8. Add salt and pepper to taste.

Serve warm over Corn Bread Stuffing on page 76 or Fluffy Mashed potatoes on page 80.

Sesame or Pumpkin Seed "Butter" (Raw)

1½ CUPS RAW SESAME SEEDS OR
    PUMPKIN SEEDS
½ CUP COLD-PRESSED CORN OR
    CANOLA OIL
2   TEASPOONS SEA SALT
½ CUP RAW AGAVE NECTAR OR RAW
    HONEY
ADDITIONAL OIL

1. Combine seeds, oil, and salt in a blender.

2. Puree at a high speed for several minutes until mixture appears smooth.

3. If needed, add extra oil by the tablespoon during blending to reach desired consistency.

4. Add sweetener and mix briefly until blended.

Use as a dip for grilled chicken or warm corn tortillas.
For a non-raw alternative, use lightly roasted seeds. This will enhance the flavor of the seed "butter."

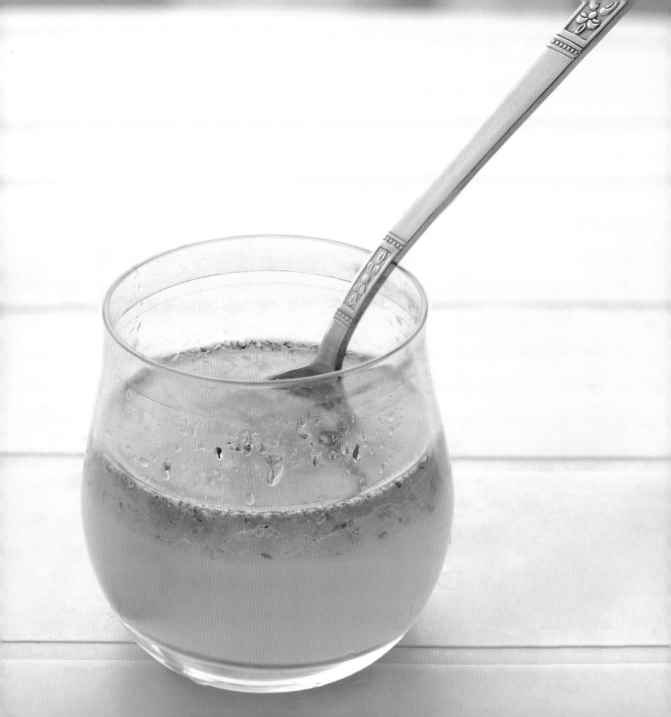

Cider-Flax Salad Dressing (Raw)

1 CUP RAW APPLE CIDER VINEGAR
½ CUP COLD-PRESSED FLAX SEED OIL
(UNFILTERED)
½ CUP RAW AGAVE NECTAR
½ TEASPOON SEA SALT

1. Combine all ingredients and blend with a whisk. Toss into salad with lettuce, raisins, cucumbers, and shredded carrots.

Citrus-Ginger Salad Dressing (Raw)

JUICE OF 1 LARGE ORANGE

¼ CUP RAW APPLE CIDER VINEGAR

3 TABLESPOONS COLD-PRESSED OLIVE OIL

1 TEASPOON FRESH GINGER, PEELED AND MINED

1 TEASPOON SEA SALT

2 TABLESPOONS RAW AGAVE NECTAR

1 TEASPOON RAW SESAME SEEDS

1. Combine all ingredients in a small mixing bowl.

2. Whisk until all ingredients are well blended.

3. Toss well into spring mix salad greens with sliced cucumber, thinly sliced carrots, and dried cranberries.

Optional: For enhanced flavor, stir in 2 tablespoons of fresh coconut milk to the salad dressing.

The Autism Cookbook

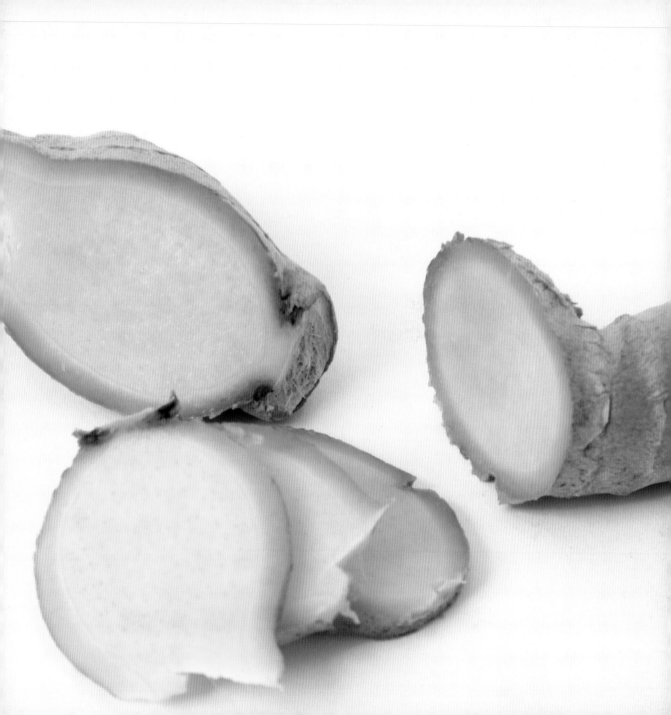

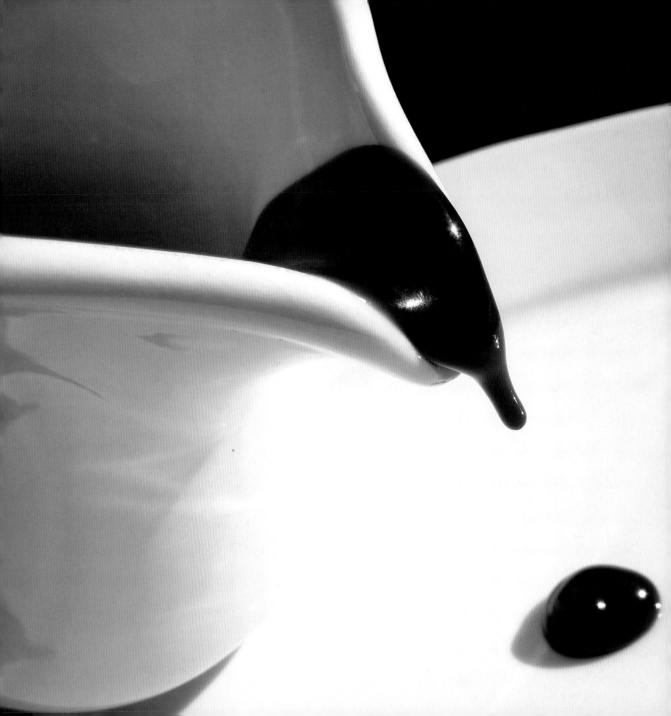

Chocolate Glaze

SWEETENER—1 CUP AGAVE NECTAR OR
2 CUPS POWDERED SUGAR
3   TABLESPOONS UNSWEETENED
COCOA POWDER
½   TEASPOON SALT

1. Combine sweetener and cocoa in a small bowl. Stir until blended.

2. If using powdered sugar, add water by the tablespoon and stir until the glaze loosens.

3. If desired, warm slightly over low heat. Stir constantly.

Spread over Brownie Bites on page 167.

Vanilla Glaze

1   CUP POWDERED SUGAR
¼   TEASPOON GLUTEN-FREE VANILLA
EXTRACT
UP TO ¼ CUP WATER

1. Place sugar in a small saucepan.

2. Add vanilla extract. Add water by the tablespoon and stir until sugar is dissolved. Do not add too much water. The glaze should resemble a thick paste.

3. If desired, warm slightly over low heat. Stir constantly.

Spread over Carrot Cake on page 168 and serve.

The Autism Cookbook

Flavored Frostings

1 CUP PALM OIL SHORTENING
SWEETENER—1 CUP AGAVE NECTAR OR
   2 CUPS POWDERED SUGAR
1 TEASPOON SALT
UP TO 3 TABLESPOONS WATER IF USING
   POWDERED SUGAR

1. Combine shortening, powdered sugar, and salt in a large bowl.

   - For vanilla flavor, add ½ teaspoon pure vanilla extract at this time.

   - For chocolate flavor, add ¼ cup unsweetened cocoa powder at this time.

   - For strawberry flavor, add 3 fresh, small strawberries at this time.

   - For lemon flavor, add juice from 1 large lemon at this time.

   - For blueberry flavor, add ¼ cup fresh blueberries at this time.

2. After adding flavor, mix at low speed with an electric mixer until frosting is smooth. If using fruit, some chunks of fruit may remain.

3. If using powdered sugar, you may add 1 teaspoon of water at a time to loosen the frosting.

Use on Vanilla Cupcakes, page 203.

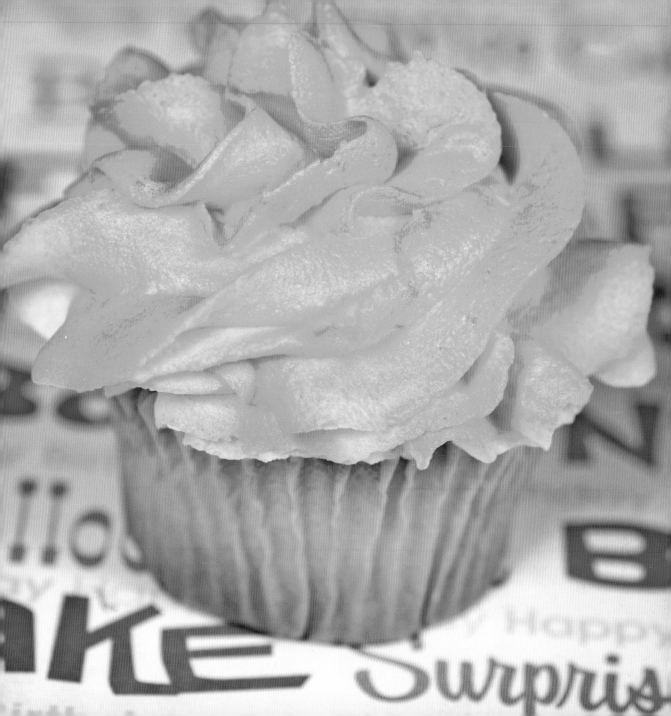

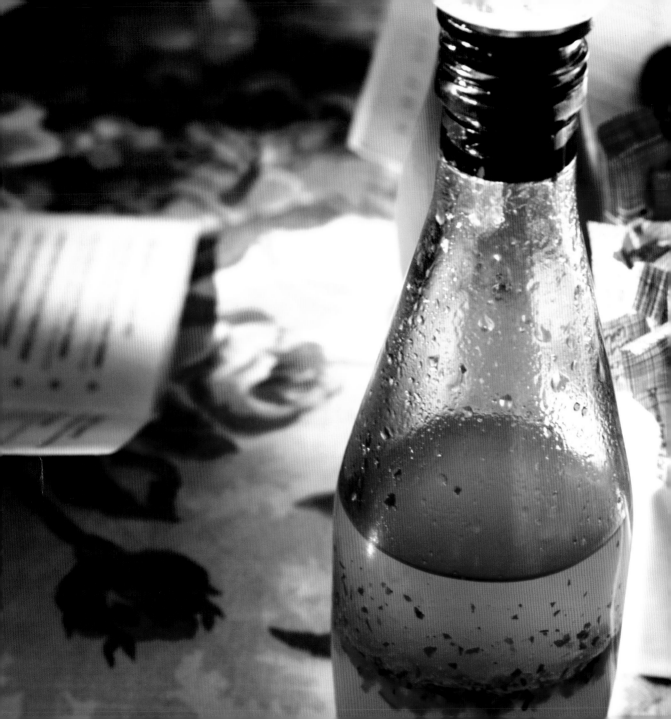

French Salad Dressing and Marinade

- ½ CUP TOMATO SAUCE (USE TOMATO PASTE FOR A THICKER DRESSING)
- ½ CUP APPLE CIDER VINEGAR
- ¼ CUP MOLASSES
- 1 TEASPOON EACH OF SALT AND ONION POWDER

1. Combine all ingredients in a mixing bowl. Whisk until well blended. Cover and keep chilled until ready to use. Use as a meat marinade or serve over salad.

French Salad Dressing and Marinade (Raw)

- 2 LARGE TOMATOES
- ½ CUP ONION, CHOPPED
- ½ CUP RAW APPLE CIDER VINEGAR
- ¼ CUP RAW AGAVE NECTAR
- 1 TEASPOON SEA SALT

1. Combine all ingredients in a blender and blend at high speed until smooth. Keep chilled until ready to use. Serve over salad greens, shredded carrots, and raisins. It can also be used as a marinade for grilling meats.

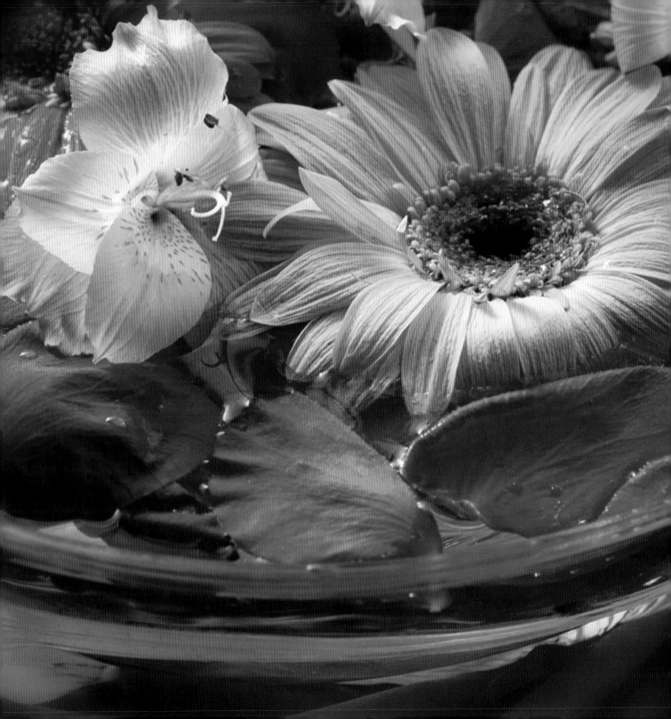

Healing Arts for Children with Autism

Human bodies have seven "chakras" that are the main energy centers of the body. They are located from the top of the head to the bottom of the torso. "Healing Arts," as named in Western society, are therapies that help balance the flow of energy in each chakra. Our cells have a constant flow of energy, which results in what we know as human life. Environmental and physical stressors can cause the energy to flow either too fast or too slow. The slower the energy moves, the more susceptible we become to illnesses and stress. An even, steady flow of energy results in increased health and feeling happy and energized.

Everyone can benefit from healing arts, especially children with autism. Balanced energy flow (or balanced chakras) results in optimal functioning throughout the whole body, which compliments the use of traditional therapies such as diet, speech, physical therapy, or ABA.

Most people cannot see the chakras with the human eye but its visibility is not necessary. The effects of balanced or off-balanced chakras can be felt. Each chakra has a corresponding physical system:

The root chakra (located at the base of the torso) corresponds to the large intestine, rectum, kidneys, and adrenal glands.
The navel chakra (located at the navel) corresponds to the reproduction system, testicles, ovaries, bladder, and kidneys.
The solar plexus chakra (located at the diaphragm) corresponds to the liver, gall bladder, stomach, spleen, small intestine, and pancreas.
The heart chakra (located at the heart) corresponds to the heart, arms, and thymus gland.
The throat chakra (located at the throat) corresponds to the lungs, throat, and thyroid gland.
The third eye chakra (located at the forehead, between the eyebrows) corresponds to the brain, face, and pituitary gland.
The crown chakra (located on the crown of the head) corresponds to the whole being and the pineal gland.

There are many Healing Art techniques (or chakra balancing techniques) including Reiki, yoga, tai chi, meditation, color therapy, visualization, and aromatherapy. In this book, I will discuss Reiki, yoga, and meditation—three essential parts of Justin's treatment plan.

REIKI

Reiki is a Japanese method for promoting healing through the laying of hands. This results in the arousing of the body's own healing response. It is a non-invasive, drug-free technique that balances the flow of energy through the body and brings harmony to the whole person. For individuals who are sensitive to touch, Reiki can be done without touching. Reiki is commonly used to enhance traditional medical therapies.

During a Reiki treatment, patients feel a warm sense of relaxation and lightness. Such deep relaxation has a positive impact on physical health, emotional health, relationships, will power, motivation, self-esteem, and more. While many people experience a cumulative effect of Reiki over several treatments, some people do report instant, life-changing experiences.

How Can Reiki Help Children with Autism?

Often, children with autism experience anxiety in social interactions and new situations. Children can also be highly susceptible to the stress and anxiety of their caregivers. Anxiety can result in problems with sleep, digestion, focus, and attention. In my experience as a practitioner, Reiki has helped children with autism to relax, sleep better, and feel more secure. While most Reiki sessions are performed while the patient is laying down, it is perfectly okay for a child to continue moving and playing while receiving a Reiki treatment. The energy will flow regardless of what the individual is doing. My son has become accustomed to laying down (and often falling asleep) during Reiki. However, I have found that allowing active children to explore works just as well. After a while, even their interactive play becomes more relaxed.

Many children on the autism spectrum face problems with "sensory integration." Sensory challenges can include over- or under-sensitivity to touch, sight, hearing, and taste. Reiki and other healing arts help us gain an awareness of our bodies in relation to space. The more comfortable we feel in the space around us, the more organized our senses flow thus, the better equipped we are to handle change and variety in sight, hearing, taste, and touch.

YOGA

Yoga is an ancient healing art originating in India. It integrates exercise, breathing, and mediation to help the person gain balance in all areas of life. Hatha yoga is one of six branches of yoga most commonly used in the West, focusing on poses.

Yoga offers countless benefits for everyone. When a series of poses are combined into a routine, the person gains increased body awareness, physical flexibility, and muscle tone. The breathing that is integrated into the routine results in relaxation and centeredness.

How Can Yoga Help Children with Autism?

Children on the autism spectrum can benefit greatly from yoga:

- Breath work results in deep relaxation, anxiety relief, focus, and some have reported reduced blood pressure and hyperactivity.
- Inverted poses provide deep pressure, which stimulates the vestibular system.
- Upward poses provide energy, alertness, and increased mood.
- All poses result in increased muscle tone, balance, and flexibility.

MEDITATION

Meditation is an awareness of inner silence. The Latin root of the word, meditation (*mederi*), means "to heal." The purpose of meditating is to achieve mental, emotional, and physical balance, which promotes healing on all levels. Meditation is beneficial for everyone, especially for parents of autistic children, helping them to find reserves of patience and energy at challenging times. More and more medical professionals are recommending meditation as an intervention for high blood pressure, heart ailments, asthma, anxiety, and insomnia.

While it does not require any specific training or teaching, meditation becomes easier with practice. When my family and I started using meditation, we found it difficult to sit quietly for even fifteen seconds. We were constantly distracted by the stimulation of the world around us and the never-ending to-do list. However, the more we practiced, the longer we were able to sit still, adding two to three minutes each week.

How Can Parents and Their Children with Autism Use Meditation?

Awareness of inner silence gives us respite from constant negative "chatter" in our subconscious minds. Stressful social encounters, physical pain, television images, and fear can feed into the "negative talk." During meditation, take the time to first become silent and as still as possible. This can be accomplished by counting ten slow breaths or by focusing on a beautiful object, such as a shiny marble. Once silent, focus your thoughts on a phrase such as, "I am healthy and safe." You can say it out loud or silently for as long as you can. If you are meditating with a child, encourage him or her to imagine something he or she loves, such as a puppy or a favorite toy. Remember that it is okay if you only get through ten seconds at a time or if your child is nonverbal and cannot repeat phrases. This is simply a guide. Keep practicing whatever "quieting" activity your child can accomplish. You will find that it will become easier and will last longer as time goes on.

Autism Resource Listing

Support Organizations and Advocacy

Talk About Curing Autism (TACANow.org)

Autism Society (www.austism-society.org)

Generation Rescue (www.generationrescue.org)

Autism Speaks (www.autismspeaks.org)

Autism Research Institute (www.autism.com)

National Vaccine Information Center (www.nvic.org)

Age of Autism (www.ageofautism.com)

Treatment Centers and Practitioners

The Brain Balance Achievement Center
  (www.brainbalancecenters.com)

Integratedenergyhealing.com (Mary Riposo)

Alternativeautismsolutions.com (Mary Riposo)

Center IMT (www.centerimt.com)

Healthy Daes Naturopathic Medical Center
  (Dr. Daemon Dae)

Trilogy Health and Wellness Center
  (Dr. Peter Bauth) (www.trilogywellness.com)

Charlie Erica Fall—Dietary Interventions for ASDs
  cefall@comcast.net.

Supplementation

Kirkman Labs (www.kirkmanlabs.com)

Nutri-West (www.nutriwest.com)

Bluebonnet (www.bluebonnetnutrition.com)

Nordic Naturals (www.nordicnaturals.com)

GFCF Grocery

Enjoy Life (www.enjoylifefoods.com)

Arrowhead Mills (www.arrowheadmills.com)

Bob's Red Mill (www.bobsredmill.com)

Kinnikinnick Foods Inc. (www.consumer.kinnikinnick.com)

Rodellevanilla.com (for gluten-free vanilla extract)

Quinoa.net

Wellshirefarms.com

Tools for Children

Lamit Bear & the Fell Better Pals (www.lamitbear.com)

Yoga Kids DVDs (www.gaiam.com)

Since We're Friends by Celest Shally

Hip Hop Baby DVDs—Candi Carter (speech and
  language development)

Baby BumbleBee DVDs (www.babybumblebee.com)

Healing Arts

National Center for Complementary and Alternative
  Medicine (www.nccam.nih.gov)

Chakras for Beginners by David Pond

Reiki for Beginners by David Vennells

Essential Reiki by Diane Stein

Toxicity Prevention and Detoxification

Ion Cleanse (www.ioncleanse.com)

BIOPRO Technology (www.bioprotechnology.com)

Other Publications

The Autism Files (www.autismfiles.com)

Glossary and Information

AGAVE NECTAR: Nectar derived from a cactus-like agave plant, used for sweetening. Its consistency and color are similar to honey.

AUTISM: A neurological disorder that affects development, communication, and social functioning. Many children with Autism have progressed considerably by eliminating gluten (from wheat, rye, and barley) and casein (from cow's milk) from their diets.

BUCKWHEAT: Buckwheat is a gluten-free plant closely related to rhubarb. Buckwheat is not related to wheat, and it is not a grain. However, buckwheat holds nutritional value that exceeds many whole grains. The seed can be finely ground to produce flour for baking or can be cooked and consumed as a side dish.

CASEIN: A protein found in cow's milk that closely resembles gluten. It provides elasticity and makes foods such as cheese, yogurt, and cow's milk "gooey."

CELIAC DISEASE: This is an autoimmune disease resulting in damage to the small intestine when gluten (from wheat, barley, or rye) is consumed. Many people who have this disease choose a casein-free diet (GFCF). It is also best to completely avoid oat. Celiac disease is not the same as wheat allergy.

CROSS-CONTAMINATION: The passing of an allergen indirectly from one source to another through improperly cleaned hands, equipment, procedures, or products.

ELIMINATION DIET: see page viii.

EMR POISONING (ELECTROMAGNETIC RADIATION): This is harmful radiation that emanates from almost all

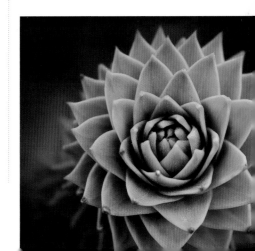

technology, electrical gadgets and radio waves. Over-exposure to radiation has been proven to cause brain tumors, hyperactivity, disease, and contamination to food, air, and water supply.

EVAPORATED CANE JUICE: A granule sweetener made from sugar cane that is less processed than traditional white, refined sugar, and therefore more nutritious. This product does not spike blood sugar as quickly as white, refined sugar.

FEINGOLD DIET: see page viii.

FLAX SEED: This is the seed of a flax plant that has multiple health benefits, including lowering cholesterol, boosting immunity, fighting constipation, and combating heart disease. It is a source of soluble and insoluble dietary fiber. The flax plant's fibers are used for clothing. Its seeds are used for food.

FOOD ALLERGY: This is an adverse reaction to a food involving the immune system. The body identifies the food as harmful and creates antibodies called IgE to fight it off. Eventually, histamines rush into the bloodstream, causing eczema, hives, sinus and throat swelling, breathing difficulty, diarrhea, a drop in blood pressure, and many other symptoms.

FOOD INTOLERANCE/ FOOD SENSITIVITY: This is an adverse reaction to a food involving the digestive system. The body has difficulty in producing sufficient amounts of digestive enzymes to break down the food. Some signs and symptoms may resemble an allergic reaction (diarrhea, vomiting, heartburn, and many other symptoms).

GLUTEN: A protein found in wheat, barley, rye, and spelt. It provides elasticity in breads, crusts, and pastries and makes foods "gooey." Oat does not contain gluten, but its protein has a very similar make up as gluten. Also, oat has a high chance for gluten contamination during its harvesting on wheat fields. Many people who wish to completely avoid gluten do not use oat products.

HEALING ARTS: A western term used to describe therapeutic activities that balance chakras, or energy flow in the body (yoga, martial arts, tai chi, meditation, Reiki). Healing arts are used to complement traditional medical care.

HISTAMINE: A chemical released by the body during an allergic reaction. Histamines are what trigger physical symptoms such as eczema, hives, sinus and throat swelling, diarrhea, drop in blood pressure, and many others.

HYPOALLERGENIC: This describes a food or substance that contains low or no amounts of common allergens, minimizing a person's chance for an allergic reaction. For example, some cosmetic or household products may omit perfumes or dyes. Some food products may omit nuts, milk, or other common allergens to lower the risk for an allergic reaction by the consumer.

IMMUNOGLOBULIN E (IgE): A type of antibody released by the immune system, primarily to protect the body from allergens. IgE signals the release of histamines that trigger physical symptoms of an allergic reaction

IMMUNOGLOBULIN G (IgG): A type of antibody released from the body when a food sensitivity culprit is consumed, triggering adverse digestive symptoms.

IONIC FOOT BATH: A warm water bath with a positively-charged magnet, used to "pull" toxins (which have a negative charge) from the body through the open pores of the feet.

MEDITATION: A soothing healing art that balances energy through quiet reflection, affirmation, breathing, and visualization.

ORGANIC: Organic crops have been grown without the use of chemicals or Genetically Modified Organisms (GMOs). Organic meats do not contain antibiotics or growth hormones. Organic foods are primarily chemical-free and processed less. Therefore, they are much easier to digest and have a higher nutritional value. See the section entitled "Going Organic" for details about organic foods.

QUINOA SEED: Quinoa is an ancient leafy plant that holds extraordinary nutritional value (including protein, essential amino acids fiber, iron, and magnesium). Like buckwheat, quinoa seeds are used to produce flour or they can be cooked in a variety of ways and eaten as a side dish.

RAW: Food is considered to be raw if it is not heated above 118°F. Fruits, vegetables, and seeds are used in this book in raw recipes. Other items used in raw recipes (not used in this book) include nuts and sprouted grains. A common method for preparing raw recipes is dehydrating. Dehydrating helps produce various textures without officially cooking the food. Cooking a food above 118°F destroys the majority of the digestive enzymes and nutrients. Including as much raw foods as possible in the diet helps improve the digestive process that gives a boost to the immune system.

REIKI: This is a non-invasive healing art that balances energy flow in the body through laying of hands.

SALICYLATES: A chemical that is either added to foods or naturally occurring in foods. It is a common culprit for sensitivity and is one of the items excluded in the Feingold Diet approach.

SPECIFIC CARBOHYDRATE DIET: see page viii.

TOXINS: Toxins are poisonous substances that have adverse effects on health. They exist in everyday living—in the commercial food supply, air, water, medicines, and even in the form of electromagnetic fields. In a healthy person, the immune system will combat poisonous substances and the digestive and excretory systems will expel them from the body.

YOGA: A healing art that balances the flow of energy in the body through movement and breathwork.

Index

The Autism Cookbook

Acknowledgments

My husband, Chris Delaine, you are my pillar of strength. Thank you so much for your undying patience and unsurpassed wisdom. Justin and Ryan Delaine, thank you for the honor of being your mother. Parents, families, and advocates of children with autism, thank you for writing this book. Children with autism, thank you for teaching the world about unconditional love.

Delaine family, Kelley family, Booker Family, Tony Lyons and Jennifer McCartney of Skyhorse Publishing, Dr. Peter Bauth, Rebecca P. Estepp (TACA), Debra N. Woodard, Mindy and Wayne Charles, Hester Bell, Yvette M. Johnson, Michele Pickett, Donna Lowry, Whole Foods Market Glastonbury, Jessica Schneider, Jackie Weaver-Bey, Donita Devance-Manzini, Chris Snell (Fayette Public Library), Charlie Erica Fall, Darren Sweeney, Carol and John Alegi, James Taylor (Fulton Public Library), Grace and Stan Simpson, Windsor Branch Library, Anika Noni Rose, Tiwanna Lewis, Kisha Cameron, Edwards Family, Stacia-Gray Crawford, ACES Autism Support Group, Southside Autism Support Group, Curtis Richardson, Karthika Siva, Annie Ong, Graciela and Tyrome Grant, The Bedford School, Spring Hill Elementary School, Ella Stoessel, Babies Can't Wait GA, Kym Kennedy, Marge Burba (Winter Growth),

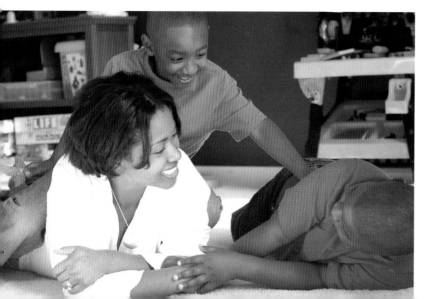

Barbara King (Hillside), Fran Wenbert and Pat Sparks of Fayette Herb Shop, Sharissa Greer, Chantal Bartley, Alread Family, Claire Cohen, Barbara Phipps, Suzanne Minarcine, Ruthan Wein, Carla Harris, David Ushery, Jeff (JJ) Johnson, New Health Nutrition Fayette staff, Oliver Family, Borcek Family, Ross Family, and to all who have contributed to the greater good and helped spread awareness of this work. Thank you!